BETTER EVERY DAY

Natural Keys to Healthy Aging

CAROL STANLEY

Table of Contents

Content

Acknowledgement

Introduction

A: Who am I and Why did I write this book ?

B: What to expect from this book.

C: A Healthy perspective.

D: The changing ways we eat.

Chapter 1: Natural Solutions for What Ails You -13
Can't Sleep, Stress and Anxiety, Feeling Tired, Skin Deep, Brain Health,
Managing Weight, Avoiding Dehydration

Chapter 2: Oils, Vitamins, Supplements, Herbs,-25 Spices and Minerals
Using Essential Oils, Benefits of Vitamins and Supplements, Herbs and Spices, Benefits of Minerals

Chapter 3: My Favorite Healthful Recipes-55
Salads & Salad Dressings, Entrees, Appetizers, Breakfast Ideas, Desserts, Easy cooking for company

Chapter 4: Homemade Health and Beauty-96

Lip balm/gloss /toothpaste/sunscreen/skin exfoliator, body butter, Face moisturizer/ shampoo/body wash, Energy Mix, Skin Mask

Chapter 5: Household Cleaning Solutions-110
Bathroom Cleaners, Kitchen Cleaners, Fruit and Veggie Wash

Chapter 6: A Wellness-Stocked Cupboard-119
Uses and benefits of: Baking Soda, Cacao Powder, Cider Vinegar, Turmeric, Coconut Oil, Hydrogen Peroxide

Chapter 7: A Grab Bag of Healthy Ideas-129
Organic Produce, Exercise, Blood pressure, Reiki, Tapping and Massage Yoga and Tai Chi, Japanese Techniques, Summing Up

Acknowledgments

This book would never have come together without my supportive husband Jim, who has stood by me through all of my various business ventures. A former burger and fries fan, he is now my partner in eating healthfully and exercising daily. Thanks go to my editor, Andrea Rouda, who coaxed my disorganized words into wonderful prose and held my hand while I was writing this book. I also want to thank all of my readers who are willing, eager and open to feeling better for the rest of their lives.

Introduction

Who I am and why I wrote this book

An artist and writer with a secret love of poker, I have no pedigrees after my name, only a lifelong passion for staying healthy. I read every responsible source about health and wellness that crosses my path and have put into action most of the ideas I share with you here. The last twenty years have been a bit frightening as I've witnessed friends and family increasing their prescription drug use, losing energy, feeling worse, gaining weight and increasing their doctor visits, causing me to wonder why this is so.

I'm no magician with a magic trick for eternal good health. But as a diligent student of nutrition and other pathways to health, a few that may be considered by some as "alternative," I have found many ways to feel good and solve some recurring issues. Having written over 500 articles on the subject of health, nutrition and medical conditions, and using the best reference sources, I have learned a lot.

The most important thing I know is not to believe everything that's out there, in books and on the Internet. Many touted solutions to every problem are totally contradictory. Thus, if I find one statement about a vitamin, mineral or supplement, I'll search for at least five reliable sources to verify that statement.

Hardly a day goes by that I do not learn something new pertaining to health issues, earning me the nickname of "medicine woman" among my friends. While I don't go around spewing unsolicited advice, I have suggested supplements, vitamins, essential oils and other healing ideas when asked. So naturally I am excited to share all my stored-up knowledge, along with my favorite recipes, with all of you. My sincere hope is that you will enjoy reading this book and use the information in it to your best advantage.

What to expect from this book

Cataloging various health conditions with healthy solutions is a good way to share my accumulated knowledge. Almost every idea I share comes from a successful outcome of a personal trial, but everyone will have a unique response to any new protocol. Also, I am not a physician so my suggestions, while valuable, should not be considered a replacement for sound medical advice from your health practitioner when needed.

Since I get so much pleasure from cooking healthful meals I have included many of my favorite recipes, featuring foods high in essential vitamins and minerals. Adding nutritious and healing spices and herbs insure that they are not only good for you but also delicious.

Before making any major changes in your life, take baby steps. Much of my advice will not change you overnight, but following it on a daily basis for a few weeks or months ultimately may bring you to your best. None of my ingredients are unduly expensive. If you swap them for your usual store-bought products and junk food, you'll see you are not spending more money by eating healthfully. And since we all react differently to foods we eat, don't experiment with vitamins, supplements, spices, herbs and essential oils without first checking with your health provider.

That caution also applies to what you put on your skin. When you lather up or slather on soaps, shampoos, creams and lotions, they enter your bloodstream rather than your digestive system. So everything that touches your skin is important and has a strong impact on your health. People often think, "Oh well, I'm just putting it on my hands, what's the harm?" The skin is a large receptor and what you innocuously smooth over your body can have a profound effect. This is one of the reasons I create many of my own skin care products and include my favorite recipes for those in this book. If you become interested in essential oils you can learn how to make your own creative brews.

A healthy perspective on aging

A fact of life is that from the moment of our birth, we begin to age. As long as we are breathing, we will continue to age. For the most part it is a slow process, and each decade brings forth new challenges and rewards. Still, for many of us, looking in the mirror on the other side of sixty can be a rude awakening. During our youth most of us are blessed with good health and great energy, getting out of bed each morning with no aches or pains. We generally don't worry about over-exposure to sun, tasking our bodies to exhaustion or eating and drinking too much.

Those who have developed healthy habits in their early years likely will enjoy a healthier aging process. And for most of us, eating good food and getting exercise was the result of someone in our life seeing to it. That's how I was raised. My mother cooked nutritious meals and made sure I played outdoors in the fresh air. I never thought of it as "must-do" exercise. I followed my mother's lead with my own kids, making most things from scratch and keeping sugar to a minimum.

At about age fifty I became more involved in lifestyle and food. I was already into whole grains, brown rice, and fresh produce, and "organic" was not yet a household word. I always made my own salad dressings and still do today. It's the smart way to go, since the recall of certain foods is an all too common event.

I cook with foods that are high in fiber as well as vitamins and minerals. I make my own sunscreen from natural ingredients, as well as other facial and body lotions.

My exercise regime has changed with aging. Through the years my husband and I have played tennis and racquetball and jogged. These days we keep fit by brisk walking or riding bikes. I also use free weights at least four times a week, meditate daily and do facial exercises.

Along with healthy eating and exercise, we both aim to keep our minds alert. To that end, I will share some wonderful nutrition ideas to boost your brainpower, along with engaging in activities like word games, Sudoku, and music. I like to think playing poker helps!

Try to enjoy each moment you can. You may not live longer following my health rules, but I feel strongly that you will feel better along the way if you eat well, exercise often and laugh a lot.

Earlier I mentioned taking baby steps. What I meant was this: Don't throw out all the food in your fridge and pantry, join an expensive gym or buy up every supplement you can on Day One. Start out slowly with the following small changes and pretty soon you will notice the difference in how you feel:

1. Start buying more fresh foods each time you shop.

2. If you have not been exercising at all, start with a walk around the block carrying two 1-pound weights for added strength.

3. Study the benefits of supplements and make sure to buy the best you can, with no preservatives.

4. Make time to prepare your own salad dressings and soups.

The changing ways we eat

The food we ate growing up was probably grown in a more healthful environment, before GMO and processed foods existed. The frozen food section was made up mostly of ice cream, vegetables and fruit. Today the frozen food section offers prepared meals for all occasions and every ethnic variety. You can eat your breakfast, lunch and dinner from a frozen selection. To keep this food tasty and fresh, a bunch of preservatives have been added. We may have eaten white bread as children, but the flour used back then was not overly processed as it is today. Mom's cooked meals "from scratch" allowed most of us to have nutritious meals prepared with fresh ingredients.

Despite the massive amount of information available today on eating healthy with whole grain, naturals and organic foods, the jury is still out as to whether or not we are actually getting healthier. Fast food options are alive and well, and judging from the many overweight kids today they are a popular option for too many families.

Dining out can be true adventure, with wildly diverse choices for meat eaters, fish lovers, vegetarians and vegans, as well as gluten-free, no-salt and no-sugar options and everything in between. But bear in mind that even the very best chefs aim to stimulate your appetite and have you return for more of their wonderful cooking. Thus restaurant food is often filled with fats, extra salt and butter, and plenty of sugar. Try not to think about that while you are out enjoying your dinner, but do think about it sometime, and plan accordingly the next time you eat out.

Chapter1: Natural Solutions for What Ails You

Most of us will have times in our lives when insomnia prevents us from enjoying a restful night's sleep. The need to lose a few pounds can feel insurmountable, bringing heavy thoughts of intense dieting. When our clothes don't fit, a frustrated feeling is imminent. We may feel tired, stressed, under the weather or just plain worried about our aging brain. There are some easy and natural solutions that can support you with each of these conditions.

Sleeplessness and insomnia

It seems that as we get older, a full night's sleep becomes more elusive. You may have trouble falling into dreamland or staying there throughout the night. Certainly, getting the noise out of our heads is often no easy feat. Our minds are racing with daily happenings, things to do and problems to solve. You can find many solutions for these problems online, or ask friends what works for them. Following are a few ideas from a variety of experts that you can do easily; hopefully one or two of them will work for you.

* Going to bed at the same time and waking up at the same time can create a sustainable sleeping pattern. This is easier said than done, especially when you are retired and don't have to be anywhere at a regular time each day. Most of us want to go bed when we want and also get up when we want. And the times of going to bed and getting up will more than likely vary from day to day. Still, it's worth remembering.

* **No TV or electronics in the bedroom will help foster sleepiness.** If you enjoy watching TV in the bedroom you will likely continue with this habit. But if you sincerely want to fall sleep sooner, you may give it a try.

* **No snacks before bedtime, especially those that contain sugar.**

* **Stop using peppermint toothpaste as it may be energizing you when you least want energy.** Also remember that toothpaste contains sugar, as well as other preservatives that may be stimulants.

Following are some suggestions that have personally worked for me:

* **Eat a small portion of a food rich in calcium or magnesium.** On a sleepless night, a tablespoon of cottage cheese has helped me relax. A banana, rich in magnesium, may also work for you.

* **Set up a diffuser filled with an essential oil in the bedroom.** Put a few drops of oil on the bottom of the feet and on wrist points, or sprinkle a little on your pillowcase. The most relaxing oils are lavender, sandalwood, lemon balm, vetiver, clary sage and sweet basil.

* Melatonin can help regulate your sleep patterns. It is actually a hormone that you can purchase over the counter, and works best as long as it is used only occasionally.

* Chamomile or any other non-caffeinated tea will relax you for sleeping. Enjoy a cup about thirty minutes before going to bed.

* Soak in a warm bath with a few drops of lavender or other calming essential oil. Follow your bath with a quiet period of meditation to help you relax further. Make sure the room is a comfortable temperature. This varies for everyone; personally I sleep best in a very cool room.

Handling stress

The amount of antidepressants and anti-anxiety medications on the market is alarming. It's obvious that stress is a natural part of life for most of us, and no matter how good your attitude may be, it is unavoidable. Sometimes it gangs up on us by teaming with anxiety. There are some solutions for temporary relief but the reality is that the issues are there and have to be dealt with, or at the very least accepted.

Never blindly buy supplements and other products you see advertised to alleviate your stress because even when they are sold over the counter, they may not be safe for you to take. If your stress persists for a prolonged period, some professional therapy may be required. Short if that, here are some easily accessible solutions to try:

* **A quick five-minute meditation might help your mind settle down.** Deep breathing for a few minutes and a brisk walk outdoors to enjoy nature will surely help. Try doing both at the same time!

* **Nutrition experts suggest that particular foods aid in calming the mind.** They include a handful of blueberries or pistachio nuts, a chunk of dark chocolate or a cup of warm tea.

* **Essential oils that lessen stress and anxiety include bergamot, vetiver, lavender, sandalwood and Frankincense.** Take note: sniffing, massaging (with a carrier oil) or diffusing are the safest ways to go with these. I keep a small bottle of lavender oil on my computer table and take a whiff every so often. While this won't solve your problems, it will create an aura of calmness.

Fatigue and lack of energy

Fatigue comes from many sources. For most of us, the

combination of inadequate sleep, too much stress and overworking our bodies and minds all add up to feeling exhausted. And don't forget that afternoon slump many of us experience. We often think a sugar-laden soft drink, some cookies or candy or a huge caffeine-injected latte will fix us up. It's true that you may get a quick boost from any one of these selections, but you'll only feel more tired when the sugar has worn off.

The best foods to eat to combat fatigue are blueberries, almonds, and a slice or two of avocado. These can give you a quick and lasting energy boost. As for supplements, doses of Vitamin C and Vitamin B12 can boost energy. I take both of these daily.

Sometimes when I get tired, a short power nap of ten to fifteen minutes revives me. If you don't have time for this try some stretches and run in place for a few minutes. A walk outside is the best remedy if you can possibly manage it.

The essential oils that can give you a punch of energy are peppermint, rosemary, bergamot, basil and geranium. You can take a quick sniff of any of these oils on a piece of cloth, or add a few drops to your bath before heading out for the day. If you apply oils directly onto the skin for a quick massage, it is best to first mix with a small amount of "carrier oil" such as coconut. You will find directions for this blend in my recipe section.

Treat your skin right

While you are nourishing your body with healthful foods, you are also nourishing your skin. When purchasing skin care products, one often thinks "the pricier the better." I have found this is not always the case.

Almost all skin products contain some preservatives to ensure freshness. Appreciating the value of natural ingredients, I make my own creams. When checking on the Internet or even watching TV advertising, you'll see that many celebrities have their own skin line. They show a bevy of beautiful *young* women with *youthful*, gorgeous skin. Then they claim their particular product will make "the appearance of wrinkles and sags" disappear. But I often wonder: will these products really do anything for *aging* skin?

Best Foods: Eating foods rich in Vitamin C aids skin health and can create the fresh look of glowing skin. All fruits and vegetables are filled with essential vitamins and water for hydration. Healthy fats such as olive oil, coconut oil and oily fish also contribute to skin health.

Best Actions: Substantial activity can create that outdoors glow. Stretching out when you sleep and preventing your face from falling into your pillow also helps prevent wrinkles. Deep breathing increases oxygen to help keep your skin looking its best. The main thing is to keep the skin moisturized as needed, especially in very dry climates. Use a sunscreen every time you go outside, even when the sun is nowhere in sight.

Best Extras for Skin, Hair and Nails: It is nearly impossible to have a perfect diet every day, so I advise taking vitamins and supplements to fill in the gaps. These should include Vitamin A, Vitamin C, Vitamin E, Vitamin D3, Folic acid, Inositol and zinc.

Best Essential Oils: All of the oils listed below will add to healthy skin. I have put together several combinations that can be found in the recipe section. Before using any oil it's always best to pre-test your skin for adverse reactions, and check ahead of time that these oils don't contraindicate any of your medications or allergies. Always use a carrier oil such as coconut oil, apricot, avocado and sweet almond.

lavender
geranium
basil
Frankincense
ylang ylang
lemongrass
cypress
tea tree (melaleuca)

Treat your brain right

The human brain is a hot topic these days. If you are an Internet addict (as I am), you will see scores of advertisements for special drinks and supplements that claim to totally eliminate dementia. But realistically, if there really were a magic bullet we would all know about it. It's still a mystery why some people have memory issues at a young age and others are still remarkably sharp well into their 80s and 90s. Is it heredity or lifestyle?

There are things you can do to improve your brain health. Exercise regularly. For example, walk four or five days a week. Or, while cleaning the house, turn up the music and do some dancing. Besides the benefits of exercise, cleaning is more fun!

Regular sound sleep and daily sun exposure are other tools in the brain-boosting arsenal. Listening to music and playing an instrument, if you are so inclined, are great pastimes, as are puzzles, memory quizzes and word or number games. They all help keep the mind active. Just like with any other organ, it's "use it or lose it."

One thing is certain: all of us worry about our brains every time we forget something. To alleviate some concern, following is a list of some of the reported best foods, vitamins and supplements for a healthy brain as well as a healthy body.

avocados
egg yolks
broccoli
celery
leafy greens
salmon
spices, especially rosemary and turmeric
coconut oil
dark chocolate
extra virgin olive oil
Vitamin B12
Vitamin D
curcumin
huperzine
phosphatidylserine
choline

Weight control

How many diets have you been on? Experts claim an 80% failure rate with most "organized" diets. I'm always sorry to see a friend lose a lot of weight and really struggle with the eating regime, just to have the pounds slowly reappear within about a year. Only an extremely small percentage of people can eat whatever they want and maintain a healthy weight.

A diet can be compared to a prison: you stay on it until you reach a desired weight and are free to go.

Unfortunately, as you slowly gain back the weight you go back to this self-imposed prison. Organized diets may offer healthy and even excellent options but you still get cravings for some of your favorite foods. Many of my friends tell me they have found the perfect diet, only to have those initial good feelings gradually and inevitably disappear.

Dining out can raise havoc with organized diets. We live in a world of food: great restaurants, TV commercials, recipes posted online, dinner parties, special occasions, and more. Resisting temptation is a daily challenge for the dieter. I have a few suggestions. They may not work for everyone, but if you are serious about losing and keeping off the weight, they could be useful.

* Be willing to change your eating habits forever, one day at a time.

* Clean out your pantry and get rid of all temptation. Throw out or give away all the sweets and carb-laden foods. If these temptations are not facing you every day, you probably won't take the time or make the effort to run out to the store to satisfy a craving.

* Fill your fridge with healthy choices, like low-carb fresh produce. Cut up fruits and veggies so you can grab some instant gratification for those hunger pangs. I rely on veggies and fruits during the day while I am home, and I'm not even trying to lose weight! If you are starving for something more

substantial, a small serving of tablespoon of cottage cheese or yogurt works wonders.

* Resist random eating like picking up a cookie here or a few nuts there. You can say "NO!" and simply walk away. Just ask yourself, "How will I feel *after* I eat that?"

* Allow yourself to splurge once a week for a special treat, then immediately return to your new, healthy way of eating.

* Exercise as much as you have time for. It will raise your metabolism, enhance your mood and keep you out of the kitchen and away from the fridge.

* Drink a lot of water to stay hydrated and also to fill you up and stave off hunger.

Dangers of dehydration

Dehydration can sneak up on you without realizing it. You will know by your symptoms whether you should head to the emergency room. This is a dangerous condition but can often be solved quickly by rehydration.

There are three grades of dehydration --mild, moderate and severe. The symptoms are easily recognizable: Diarrhea, vomiting, dizziness, dry mouth and general weakness. Sometimes if you recognize the symptoms of mild dehydration soon enough and start sipping water, especially water containing electrolytes, you can head off some of the more debilitating symptoms.

Especially as we age, most people are often mildly dehydrated. The problem is that we use our feeling of thirst to tell if we are properly hydrated, and it doesn't always give an accurate reading. Living in a dry climate will exacerbate dehydration. I thought eating lots of produce would eliminate the problem, but after having a dehydration attack that landed me in the emergency room, I now drink at least a quart and half of water daily. It is easier to accomplish this than you think. Keep your water bottle handy and sip throughout the day. You'll be amazed at how quickly the water will disappear.

If you keep up your water intake on a daily basis you will not need to consume water with electrolytes, like a Gatorade type of drink. If you are very physically active you will need to drink during your workout to stay adequately hydrated.

Chapter 2 : The Essential Extras

Essential oils

Essential oils have been around for thousands of years and are even mentioned in the Bible. Before prescription drugs were common, essential oils were blended and used for many medical conditions. There are hundreds of essential oils, and almost as many conditions that they can help.

I love using essential oils and especially experimenting with my own blends. To create them, I have spent a lot of time researching which particular oils work best together, and in what amounts. The Internet is rife with differing opinions about these oils, with self-proclaimed experts fearlessly claiming to have "magically" cured many diseases and conditions with them. Not all of them have merit. The oils that I write about have proven results that I stand by. I have my favorites and will share with you the top 20.

A quick and important reminder is that many of us will have different results, thus you should become your own "expert" on what works best for you. Have some fun and experiment with various oils to see what you can determine. Always check to make sure that the oils you choose do not interfere with your prescriptions and even any of the over-the-counter supplements you consume. Test the oil on a small area on your skin for any adverse reaction.

Keep in mind that these oils are powerful and should be used judiciously. All essential oils are very concentrated, and a small amount goes a long way. For example, just one drop of essential lemon oil uses at least one pound of lemons, and each drop of lavender oil requires one pound of lavender plant to produce.

It's important to buy high quality essential oils. If the bottle says there is added fragrance or preservatives, the oil is not pure. The bottle must be made of a dark-colored glass, for example amber or green. You can choose the organic kind if you wish. I have used both and always buy brands I recognize.

Essential oils are excellent for a variety of different conditions. Besides that, just their pleasant scents and relaxing qualities are almost reason enough to incorporate them into your normal health and beauty routine. Oils are commonly used for relief of muscle or joint pain and as an ingredient in facial creams, skin lotions, toothpaste and sunscreen. They also help with relaxation and sleeping, stress reduction, increased energy and enhanced alertness. Lastly, many of them are a great addition to cleaning solutions used in the home.

Here are several effective ways to use oils:

As a Massage: Always dilute any oil with a carrier oil to lessen its strength. Take a small amount of the oil combination and gently massage into your skin. For quick results, the best places to massage are on the bottom of the feet, behind the ears and on the inside of the wrists.

As a Scent: Use a diffuser and allow the unique scent to permeate your room for several hours before bedtime. The essential oils create a warm atmosphere, and this action will greatly help to create calmness and assist in falling asleep easily. There are many diffusers available online and all of them are easy to use. Simply fill the container with a few drops of your favorite oil and a small amount of water. I love that aroma of lavender wafting in the air as I am falling asleep. If you're feeling tired, stressed or restless, inhale the oil directly by applying some to a thin piece of cotton. I do this often when I need a quick burst of energy.

For Ingestion: There are many medicinal uses for essential oils but since I am not a doctor or scientist I cannot endorse using essential oils to cure a major health issue. Your research will assist you in making such decisions. Personally, I am not a fan of taking these oils orally, nor do I recommend adding essential oils to your foods or using directly on your skin. A few of the oils are toxic when ingested, while others may not mix well with medicines and vitamins you may be using.

Carrier oils

Carrier oils work well to dilute the strength of the essential oils, ending up with a solution that is approximately 10% essential oil to 90% carrier oil. Here are some of the more popular carrier oils:

coconut oil
avocado oil
apricot kernel oil
sweet almond oil
jojoba oil
olive oil

Following are brief descriptions of my favorite essential oils. I hope you will be inspired to read more about all of them and eventually find your own favorites.

Lavender Essential Oil: My favorite of all, this one has more uses than other essential oils. Lavender smells delightful and can help you relax and improve your mood. It is also effective in healing cuts and wounds, and is compatible with many other oils. Sometimes as we age, our level of stress increases. This is certainly true for me. Because of that, there are times when I take a whiff of lavender oil right from the bottle and my stress begins to dissipate immediately.

Eucalyptus Essential Oil: If you've used chest rubs you will immediately recognize the scent of eucalyptus. It is great help for relieving symptoms of bronchitis and other allergies, as well as a variety of other common aches and pains.

Frankincense Essential Oil: This oil is useful for many conditions. Used during Biblical times for a variety of ceremonies, it has an earthy, woody scent. Its healing properties make it a popular choice for skin conditions. When used regularly, it has reportedly lightened those pesky "age spots." The pleasant scent of Frankincense creates a warm and relaxed feeling. Just a few drops in your favorite lotion can help lessen skin dryness and irritation, which is why I add Frankincense to some of my skin moisturizer and stress recipes. This oil is also known to aid digestion and calm stomach issues. Because there are some known allergies to this oil, be sure to ask your health provider about whether it is safe for you.

Ginger Essential Oil: Ginger has a strong, pleasant scent and mixes well with many other essential oils. If you already use ginger in your cooking you more than likely will not have any problem applying it to your skin. As with other essential oils, a few drops go a long way. Ginger is widely recognized for its anti-nausea properties. Personally I have found that putting few drops on my wrists helps calm an upset stomach. The basic ingredient of ginger is *gingerol*, an anti-inflammatory helpful in keep the body in balance. Warnings: Avoid contact around eyes and inner ears and do not use when pregnant or nursing.

Lemon Essential Oil: Along with its refreshing lemon scent, this oil has rejuvenating and energizing properties. It is touted to help inflammation, promote healthy blood circulation and improve cardiovascular health. The oil is best diluted with a carrier oil and massaged into the skin. Again, please test a little bit on your skin to make sure there is no reaction. Pour a small amount onto a clean cloth and inhale, and you will feel energized. Adding a few drops to your cleaning solutions will help clean more thoroughly. Warning: It is possible to have sensitivity in the skin and respiratory system, so check with your health provider before using. Do not use lemon oil on your skin when heading out into direct sunlight, or if you are pregnant or nursing.

Bergamot Essential Oil: This oil has a spicy, citrus scent. Citrus scents are very pleasant to use and energize and relieve temporary stress. Applied directly on the skin with a carrier oil, its healing benefits will help with fungal infections. Bergamot is often added to blends that relieve anxiety and stress. This oil is also best not used in direct sunlight. Actually, all citrus type essential oils are best not used outdoors in sunlight. Bergamot is said to help regulate your cardiovascular system, although I suggest checking with your health provider before using it for your health issues.

Oregano Essential Oil: Many of us know and use oregano as a common cooking spice that adds a lot of flavor to a variety of cuisines. But did you know that oregano is also known for its antibiotic qualities? Topically it can help with fungus infections, although this claim is still under debate. Oregano also has many cardiovascular benefits. Inhaling it when blended with steaming water can relieve sinus infections and stuffy noses.

Before investing in this oil, check with your health provider as some people are allergic to oregano. If you are allergic to the spice you will probably also be allergic to the essential oil. Put a small, diluted drop on your skin and check for any adverse reactions. I am convinced that when I use this oil regularly it staves off infections and even ordinary colds.

Peppermint Essential Oil: Peppermint comes from the peppermint plant and has its familiar aroma. Use it sparingly. Very often a quick sniff will open your sinuses and you will feel immediately energized. Peppermint can be very therapeutic for stomach issues and a variety of other physical ailments. Be sure to mix it with a carrier oil as it is very strong when undiluted.

I add peppermint to my homemade toothpaste and even store-bought cleaning solutions. As we age our teeth easily discolor and mine are a lot whiter since using my own toothpaste. My husband goes to the dentist every three months for a deep cleaning. It took me a while to convince him, but I finally got him to try my homemade version. The hygienist was pleasantly surprised and asked what he had done differently on his teeth, since for the first time she didn't have to do a deep cleaning. I happily took full credit for that!

Do not use peppermint if you are pregnant or nursing, and on young children under the age of seven. Peppermint is a natural stimulus and could cause rashes, variation in breathing, pain, nausea, urinary problems and even convulsions. Diabetics should not use this oil as it could trigger a lowering of blood sugar.

Rosemary Essential Oil: Rosemary has a clean, refreshing herbal smell. If you already use the herb for cooking you will enjoy this oil for massage or diffusing. It is touted to create clarity, relieve coughs for several hours and relieve headaches. Add a little carrier oil and massage some onto your pets for a shinier, healthier coat. Rosemary is often added to shampoos and conditioners to stimulate hair growth and even control dandruff. It is also good for stress; just a drop of oil on a cloth and a good sniff can help lower your stress level.

Pregnant women, nursing mothers and children under 10 should not use this oil. The same goes for those who suffer from epilepsy or high blood pressure. Avoid contact with the eyes, ears and nose. Rosemary is very strong by itself, so it is best used with a carrier oil.

Tea Tree Essential Oil: Also known as *melaleuca oil*, it has many uses. Known for its anti-fungal, antibacterial and antiseptic qualities, it has a slightly medicinal scent. Having this all-purpose oil on hand is a good idea for many common conditions including bacterial infections, open wounds and minor skin abrasions.

Other uses of tea tree oil are as a toothbrush cleaner, laundry freshener, and even for pest control. Unless prescribed, this oil is not to be ingested. Instead, massage with carrier oil or add to a diffuser to inhale, which can help alleviate cold symptoms. A few drops applied to a minor cut or scrape will help avoid infection.

Sandalwood Essential Oil: Recognized for its exotic lingering scent, I enjoy opening the bottle and getting a quick whiff. The scent has a calming effect and is often used commercially in perfumes and creams. Mixing sandalwood with a carrier oil soothes rashes, scar tissue and other skin ailments. I often add a few drops to my regular conditioner as it adds luster to dry hair.

Thyme Essential Oil: Many of us are familiar with thyme as a cooking spice we add to a variety of dishes. As with many essential oils, it has antibacterial, anti-fungal and anti-virus properties. It is also used in hair and beauty products and in mouthwash. It is touted to help prevent hair loss and keep aging skin at its peak.

Sweet Marjoram Essential Oil: The scent is spicy and fresh. Like many essential oils, it can help relieve stress and control anger. It is said to relieve joint and muscle pain. Marjoram is a popular herb used in a variety of culinary dishes. This oil mixes well with many other oils. The usual warnings apply: It is best used with a carrier oil, sampled on your skin prior to use, and never ingested.

Clary Sage Essential Oil: Clary sage has a potent, nutty scent. It is commonly used for vision problems including tired and irritated eyes. Commercially, it is an ingredient in soaps, detergents, lotions and creams. This oil can be used for insomnia, stress, and back pains when added to blends with carrier oils. As an herbal product it is found in many herbal compounds. Warnings: Clary sage is considered safe but should not be used in combination with alcohol or drugs. People with low blood pressure should not use it.

Roman Chamomile Essential Oil: Roman chamomile has a warm and slightly fruity scent. It is often added to shampoos, lotions and other beauty products. It has a positive effect on a variety of digestive problems and skin ailments. Known to sooth skin burns and diaper rash when added to either baby cream or carrier oils, this oil is best used as a massage or infusion. It blends well with many oils such as lemon, clary sage, bergamot and lavender. Warnings: Many people who are allergic to different plants will have an allergic reaction to Roman chamomile. Be sure to blend it well with a carrier oil.

Neroli Essential Oil: It takes 1,000 pounds of oranges to make one pound of neroli oil. Its pleasing scent is added to many perfumes. Used to relieve fever and banish nervousness in Biblical times, today it is alleged to help alleviate depression, aid circulation and calm headaches. Neroli is also useful in the treatment of skin irritations. It is best tolerated with a carrier oil. Warnings: Do not use this oil on young children or pregnant women. It occasionally can create either a restless feeling or drowsiness.

Geranium Essential Oil: With a wonderful sweet scent and no known irritating qualities, this oil is uplifting and can be therapeutic for skin conditions and dry skin. While it will not totally rid you of stress and depression, geranium can lighten your spirits temporarily. I have blends for a facial moisturizer and a body cream scented with geranium. Geranium mixes well with many other oils. You can make a natural deodorant by combining several drops of geranium oil with half a cup of water in a spray bottle.

Vetiver Essential Oil: This is another favorite of mine. It has a unique grassy scent and is helpful in promoting sleep and calming restlessness. In experiments with children with ADHD, vetiver has been found successful in creating a sense of calmness. Added to other oils, it aids in reducing foot pain. It is a common ingredient of many popular perfumes.

Ylang Yiang Essential Oil: With its flowery banana scent, this oil is used to relieve tension and is sometimes called "the woman's oil." Topically massaged into the scalp, it will help revitalize dry and lifeless hair. This oil is known for its ability to create calmness, either by inhaling it directly from the bottle or using in a diffuser. Warnings: This oil can cause irritation, such as headaches and nausea, if over-used. Like all essential oils, less is best.

Vitamins and minerals

The vitamins, minerals and supplements I have selected are the ones that I currently use or have used in the past and are among the most common ones taken. There are literally hundreds of vitamin, mineral and supplement combinations on the market today so it is easy to get overly zealous when experimenting with them. Taking supplements should not be a substitute for healthy eating, although they can often fill in the gaps. Some of my chosen supplements are valuable for specific conditions and others are used to prevent conditions from developing.

As we age, so do our immune systems, causing us to become more susceptible to diseases and uncomfortable conditions. It is wise to do some research concerning what is available to help your particular issues. If you have friends who are into supplements, ask them what they take. I generally suggest taking vitamins and supplements that contain only one vitamin or mineral. A multi-vitamin often can have either too little or too much of any one vitamin or mineral, and it may be just the one you need the most, or the least!

I am always super-cautious when suggesting how much or how often someone should take any supplement, vitamin or mineral. There is so much written about all of this, and it is ultimately up to each individual to find the specific formula to reach his or her best potential. The first step is to streamline any diet down to eating all fresh foods. Loading up with supplements won't do the trick. A friend of mine takes about 30 different supplements a day but eats whatever he wishes, be it good or bad. The outcome for him is not yet known, but I believe that eating conscientiously, with the addition of a few well-selected supplements, will result in overall better health in our later years.

Vitamin A: Food Sources: Milk, eggs, carrots, leafy greens and fortified cereals. Vitamin A promotes healthy eyes, skin and hair and supports your immune system. This is a vitamin with dosage limits. Chances are if you eat enough produce you will be getting your daily requirement.

Vitamin B1 (Thiamine): Food Sources: Beans, whole grains and fortified cereals, pork, beef, poultry, nuts. Helps process carbohydrates and strengthens the immune system. It is water-soluble, so the body does not store it. It is unusual to be deficient in this vitamin, except in some rare cases and with certain diseases.

Vitamin B2 (Riboflavin): Food Sources: Milk, bread, almonds, asparagus, dark meat chicken, beef, mushrooms, shellfish and oily fish. Vitamin B2 is not lost during cooking. It supports many body processes and helps create red blood cells. This vitamin helps regulate thyroid acuity, proper growth and energy production.

Vitamin B3 (Niacin): Food Sources: Poultry, whole grains, mushrooms, tuna, green peas, grass-fed beef and peanuts. An aid to digestion, B3 also regulates cholesterol and thus is helpful in treating heart disease. It is often prescribed for a variety of cardiovascular concerns and the dosage must be regulated due to possible negative side effects.

Vitamin B6: Food Sources: Potatoes with skin, white meat chicken and turkey, eggs, peas, beef and spinach. Supports the nervous system and helps break down sugars stored in the body. It also supports adrenal function and key metabolic processes.

Vitamin B12: Food Sources: Beef, clams, mussels, crabs, salmon, poultry and some foods that have been fortified with this vitamin. Vitamin B12 is water-soluble so it is not stored in the body. It is essential for healthy skin, hair and nails and supports the digestive system and the nervous system. It also has an energizing effect.

Vitamin D: Food Sources: Fortified cheeses, milk, cereals, egg yolks, salmon and cod fish. In the past several years there has been much hype in the news about the value and importance of vitamin D. Vitamin D can be found easily outdoors, in sunlight. It has a role in supporting healthy bones and teeth, as well as the immune system, brain and nervous system.

This vitamin regulates insulin, supports cardiovascular health and helps regulate the amount of calcium in your body. While there is some evidence that it staves off a variety of diseases, it can interact negatively with some medications so check with your health provider before starting a regimen of vitamin D.

Vitamin E: Food Sources: Leafy greens, almonds, mangos and pistachio nuts. Vitamin E serves the body in many areas such as cardiovascular and brain support. Getting this vitamin from food is the best way to go. If you are taking blood thinners, check with your health provider before taking a vitamin E supplement, as it has been known to be a natural blood thinner. Topically it restores dull hair, is great for skin problems and strengthens nails.

Folate (B9): Food Sources: Fortified cereals and other grain products, beans and dark leafy greens. This is essential for pregnant women because it helps to regulate the growing baby's vitals. It also regulates cholesterol and blood pressure and aids in colon health.

Vitamin K: Food Sources: Dairy products, leafy greens, fortified products such as orange juice and milk. Its benefits include its blood-clotting ability and help in maintaining healthy bones.

Minerals

Calcium: Food Sources: Most dairy products, leafy greens, broccoli, and sesame seeds. Many fortified foods are enhanced with calcium. One tablespoon of sesame seeds provides up to 35 percent of your daily calcium requirement. You often find this vitamin in supplements containing both calcium and magnesium. Calcium keeps bones and teeth strong. It also protects the heart muscles and helps to normalize blood pressure.

Chromium: Food Sources: Broccoli, barley, beans and oats. Fortunately the need for this mineral is minimal as it appears in only small amounts in the body. Still, it is important for health issues such as high blood pressure and regulating blood sugar.

Copper: Food sources: Sesame seeds, cashews, beef liver, crab, oysters, mushrooms, lentils, almonds and dark chocolate. An essential trace mineral found in the liver, brain, heart, kidneys and skeletal system, it is helpful with cognitive function, motor skills and bone strength. Only small amounts are needed to reap its benefits.

Magnesium: Food sources: Pumpkin seeds, spinach, Swiss chard, cashews, black beans, avocados and sesame seeds. Magnesium is the body's most essential mineral. Most people only get about half of what is needed to maintain good health. Strong bones, blood sugar levels and blood pressure are just a few of the areas influenced by the amount of magnesium you take in. There are a wide variety of different types of magnesium available and only a few are truly beneficial.

Magnesium oil is a good option for supplying yourself with enough magnesium. Another option is using a magnesium oil spray daily. The best place to spray is the bottom of your feet where our nerve receptors are close to the surface of the skin. I put some on before turning in at night and it helps me fall asleep, happy to know I am getting a good dose of magnesium.

Manganese: Food sources: Pumpkin seeds, spinach, Swiss chard, cashews, black beans, cashews, avocados and sesame seeds. You may overlook this one when you think of minerals in general since our bodies need just a small amount. However it is essential in fighting free radicals, and indirectly helps control blood sugar levels.

Molybdenum: Food sources: Legumes, leafy greens, liver, lentils and peas. This is another mineral that many people know nothing about. Molybdenum acts as a catalyst of enzymes and is important in the breakdown of certain amino acids. It is rare to have a deficiency in this mineral.

Phosphorous: Food sources: Sunflower seeds, white beans, tuna, turkey breast, almonds, brown rice, broccoli and eggs. Phosphorous is important to most organs in the body. It helps regulate hormones naturally, helps muscles to contract, and regulates heartbeat rhythms. It is also a factor in avoiding tooth decay.

Potassium: Food sources: Spinach, bananas, acorn squash, salmon and avocados. There are many symptoms of poor health related to low levels of potassium. This important mineral helps regulate blood pressure, discourage kidney disorders and strengthen heart muscles. Another benefit: it helps keep the body hydrated.

Selenium: Food sources: Turkey, chicken, scallops, beef, Brazil nuts, cabbage and spinach. It is thought to help stave off different types of cancer, defend against heart disease, prevent viruses, support the thyroid and insure a strong immune system. As with many vitamins and minerals, it is best to get your selenium from foods rather than from a supplement.

Zinc: Food sources: Cooked oysters, beans, wheat germ, spinach, pumpkin seeds and cashews. Zinc assists in creating proper growth, healing of wounds and thyroid function. The supplements have been reported to have a variety of negative side effects, so it is best to get zinc from the foods you eat. Required amounts differ according to age and gender, so check with your doctor or pharmacist.

Supplements

After you gain some knowledge of vitamins and minerals, the next step in your education is an understanding of supplements. There are many available supplements for different conditions and knowing what to take can be daunting. You will get advice from everyone pertaining to things they have tried and found to work, or else have failed. Again, we are all different and sometimes our particular aches and pains as well as other challenging symptoms can seemingly disappear spontaneously without any help from us.

Every month when my new Swanson catalog arrives, I go through it carefully. This company has grown through the years and now carries a variety of brands of vitamins, minerals and supplements, as well as organic foods, essential oils, coffee, pet products and more. It is so important to do your homework and become familiar with the many products on the market.

I am a big fan of natural products, but they also can have some negative side effects. And mixing and matching doesn't always work! So be judicious and get professional advice before buying a lot of natural healthful products and all those healthy-sounding vitamins, minerals and supplements.

Many vitamins and minerals do support the following health issues. The ones I list here are supplements for specific conditions.

Bilberry: Bilberries are similar to blue berries in appearance and taste. You don't commonly see this berry at the grocery store, but the supplement supports many eye issues. It is reported to improve night vision, circulation problems, It is best not to take if you are taking blood thinners.

Astaxanthin: Several sources report this to be "the supplement of the century" and valuable in treating many conditions. The main food containing astaxanthin is wild-caught salmon, and the redder the better. Another natural source is green algae. As an antioxidant it is reportedly stronger than vitamin C. Some studies have found it helps rid the body of inflammation.

Lutein and Zeaxanthin: Both of these supplements support good eyesight, and can act as a preventative measure against developing Age-related Macular Degeneration (AMD), or slowing down its progression if you already have it. In some cases it has been known to cause AMD to backtrack and disappear completely. Certainly learn more about it if you have eye issues. Some natural sources of these supplements are flaxseed, pumpkin seeds, walnuts, spinach, kale and egg yolks.

You may want to add a specific eye vitamin to ensure getting all the necessary nutrients to support your vision. Years ago my husband was diagnosed with the beginning stages of macular degeneration. He has now been taking lutein and zeaxanthin for about 10 years, and the problem has all but disappeared.

Alpha Lipoic Acid: Some foods that contain alpha lipoic acid are broccoli, yams, tomatoes, Brussels sprouts, carrots and red meat. This supplement is reported to regulate your blood sugar, fight inflammation and slow the aging process. It helps activate glutathione in your body and can relieve neuropathy.

Ginseng: Although it is an herb, ginseng is also available in a variety of combination supplements. Its natural anti-inflammatory properties make it useful for treating several different ailments, such as regulating blood sugar. It is most easily found and best consumed in a wide range of teas.

Beetroot Powder: This is one of the latest sensational supplements out there to add to your repertoire. I add two scoopfuls to water and sip it during the day. It is reported to increase stamina and keep your blood pressure at healthy number. It has lowered both my diastolic and systolic readings several points. Beets increase the nitric oxide in your blood, so it stands to reason that if you eat a large portion of beets you will get the same results. (This is not true for sweet pickled beets.)

Glutathione: This supplement is found in every cell in the body. Glutathione is helpful in lowering some types of high blood pressure. If you are under prolonged stress your natural glutathione will be reduced. Many people have been running out to buy the synthetic version, but many medical experts feel that has little value. A diet rich in organic produce helps produce glutathione and greatly enhance your internal health, but be aware that cooking the vegetables reduces its inherent value by approximately half. Whey protein is the best product to take to keep your glutathione working properly for your body.

Coenzyme Q10: Food Sources: Beef, poultry, fatty fish, peanuts, fruits, vegetables, sesame seeds, and pistachio nuts. This is naturally produced in our bodies but tends to diminish as we age. The newer and more popular version is called *Ubiquinol*, which is reported to be more bio-available. This means there is a higher proportion of the active ingredient entering the bloodstream, making it more powerful and effective. It also supports good cardiovascular health.

Lycopene: A bright red carotene and carotenoid found in watermelon, tomatoes, tomato juice, pink grapefruit and papaya. Besides its cardiovascular benefits, it supports prostate health. Lycopene is often included in supplements containing several other supplements. Because there are a few warnings related to lycopene, check with your health provider before doing any experimenting.

L Carnitine: This is found mostly in red meat, pork, chicken and dairy products. It is beneficial to heart health and also plays a part in reducing fatigue and assisting in weight loss. L Carnitine is available in supplements that also include *taurine*.

Herbs and spices

Most of us commonly cook with a variety of herbs and spices and never give a thought to the great health benefits they add. Until I began studying the science behind herbs and spices I simply added them to a variety of dishes during cooking. Once you learn about them you will feel even better about flavoring your food, knowing you are doing your body a favor as well as your taste buds.

It is difficult to explain the various flavors of many herbs and spices, as they are all so unique. Over time you will develop your favorites to use for general cooking. As the name implies, they really do spice up your food! Many spices and herbs are found in teas, tinctures and essential oils.

Herbs and spices come from different parts of a particular plant. An herb is the green, leafy part, whereas a spice can come from the root, stem, seed, fruit, flower or bark of the tree or plant. A plant can be host to both an herb and spice at the same time; a good example is cilantro and coriander.

You may grow your own spices and herbs or use the dry version, the most popular for ease and shelf life.

Having an herb garden is a fun hobby and provides you with fresh herbs, always superior in taste and texture.

Basil: A favorite spice for many people, it is often associated with tomatoes as the two go so well together. This spice is popular in Italian dishes as well as casseroles and salads. Basil, rich in vitamins and minerals, is appreciated for its antibacterial qualities. I found I was purchasing a lot of basil as I use it just about every day, so I wised up and started growing my own in a pot right outside my kitchen door.

Bay Leaf: The adventurous cook often drops in a few bay leaves to soups, casseroles and sauces. Bay leaves possess lots of vitamins, potassium and zinc.

Cardamom: This is a traditional spice to use in baked goods such as cakes and pies, as well as many Indian dishes. It is considered to be anti-inflammatory and improve circulation. It's also loaded with vitamin C, magnesium, potassium and zinc, and contains lots of fiber.

Cayenne Pepper: This wonderful spice tastes great and adds some heat to your food. It is an anti-inflammatory and thus helps your gut health and your circulation. It contains a healthy amount of B vitamins, vitamin A and magnesium. If you like hot food, knowing that cayenne will keep your gut healthy as you age is a bonus!

Cinnamon: A variety of foods including baked goods, fruit, sauces and of course cinnamon toast benefit from this popular spice that also helps regulate blood sugar. It contains fiber and manganese and thus is also an aid to digestion. I often add this spice to soups and salad dressings, just to make things interesting.

Clove: Along with its unique flavor, clove has some therapeutic value. When mixed with honey it can ease a toothache or calm an upset stomach. It adds flavor to pork and ham dishes, hot drinks and baked items. Cloves mix well with cinnamon and nutmeg and add dimension to cooked fruit.

Coriander/ Cilantro: Despite their differences, coriander comes from the seeds and cilantro from the leaves of the same plant. Cilantro is commonly used to flavor many salsas and Mexican dishes, while the coriander seeds are a valuable addition to soups, salads and curries. Combine some chopped cilantro with sour cream for a healthy dip that contains Vitamin K and potassium and helps strengthen bones.

Cumin: Another popular spice for Mexican dishes, soups and stews, a dash of cumin delivers a pungent taste to chili and curry dishes. Cumin contains vitamin B and is an aid to digestion.

Dill Weed: This popular pickling spice also does wonders for egg salad, tuna salad, most soups and a variety of cheese dishes. Dill aids digestion and is rich in vitamins and minerals.

Fennel: A fresh fennel bulb, with its distinct licorice flavor, resembles celery in looks but not in taste. I use the dry spice along with other herbs in making curry dishes. It contains dietary fiber, acts as a diuretic and can help neutralize stomach acid. Fennel tea is great for settling an upset stomach and easing constipation.

Fenugreek: This member of the bean family has been used therapeutically for hundreds of years. Filled with vitamins and minerals, it is effective in treating stomach disorders and respiratory issues. It is a popular ingredient for many Indian dishes and curries, and both the seeds and leaves can be used. It has a tangy, slightly bitter burnt sugar taste. As with most foods, check with your health provider to make sure it is compatible with any drugs or vitamins you may be taking.

Garlic: Most of us love garlic though it often does not love us back in the "bad breath" department! This little bulb enhances many dishes, adding flavor and depth. It is reportedly a great boost for the immune system, containing anti-bacterial properties as well as lots of vitamins and minerals.

Ginger: Widely known for its anti-nausea support, ginger is helpful before a long car ride or boat ride if you are susceptible to motion sickness. I use grated or shaved ginger in many sauces, curries, and stir-fries. It has lots of vitamins, minerals, and vitamin B complex.

Marjoram: Marjoram is one of those spices you can just sprinkle here and there. It enhances cheese dishes and vegetable casseroles, and creates a tasty combo with oregano, thyme and basil. It also aids digestion, creates a feeling of calmness and is loaded with vitamins and minerals.

Nutmeg: A popular spice around the winter holidays, it is often used as a topping on eggnogs and in pumpkin pies. It's also great in curries, meat dishes and many other baked dishes. Use it sparingly as the flavor is strong, so a little goes a long way. Nutmeg supports a healthy digestive system and is said to support brain health.

Oregano: There are several types of oregano, so if you have a green thumb you might want to experiment with a few. It grows easily and you'll always have some handy to spice up your cooking. (We have a patch of it in our yard and the more I use, the more it grows.) Its unique flavor is integral to Italian and Mexican dishes. Oregano is used frequently for respiratory issues and also aids digestion. Many farmers are now using oregano for their animals in lieu of traditional antibiotics.

Paprika: Everyone knows paprika for its bright red color. The addition of this colorful spice to pale meats such as pork and chicken ups their visual appeal. It has a mild flavor but still adds that extra pizzazz. Besides that, it contains beneficial vitamins and minerals.

Peppermint: An ingredient in many products that we use besides foods, like mouthwash and toothpaste, the flavor and scent of peppermint scent are instantly recognizable. The leaves are often added to ice tea, salads and chutneys. An extra benefit is gained from its considerable vitamins and minerals.

Rosemary: I love the aroma of rosemary cooking, especially on roasted chicken. It lends a unique flavor to meat, pork, lamb and many veggies. This spice blends well with many other spices. It is an anti-inflammatory that aids digestion and circulation and a host of other conditions.

Sage: Widely used in turkey and other poultry stuffing recipes, sage enhances the flavor of meat dishes, soups and grains. The sage leaf is often used in medicines. It aids digestion and there is some newer speculation that it supports brain health.

Savory: A tasty spice that adds flavor to fish and meat dishes as well as vegetarian and grain dishes. Savory has a healthy amount of fiber and Vitamin C. It is widely used in its powder form.

Tarragon: If you've ever had Béarnaise sauce you've had this aromatic herb, popular in meat dishes and herb butters. It contains antioxidants and minerals, as well as vitamins A and C. It is considered an herb as the leaves are used.

Thyme: Another versatile spice for meat and vegetables and part of many Mediterranean dishes, thyme can lessen sore throat pain and ease coughs and colds. It's also a diuretic, effectively treats athlete's foot, and benefits skin and hair.

Turmeric: This multi-faceted spice fights inflammation, offers brain support and helps aching muscles. Also referred to as *curcumin*, it lends its yellow color to curry blends. (Its natural yellow color can leave permanent stains, so avoid getting it on your clothes.) For the most benefit, there should be a large percentage of *curcumin* in the blend you purchase. Check to be sure as many blends on the market contain only a small amount. Purchase a well-known brand, preferably organic. I use fresh, raw turmeric root in cooking, blending it with black pepper or combining with organic turmeric powder to create curries.

Chapter 3: My Favorite Healthful Recipes

Besides the delicious ingredients, within each of the following recipes there's a good share of vitamins, minerals and fiber. They are all flexible, allowing you to add other spices or veggies and still get great results, particularly with the soups and salads. I find it challenging to follow recipes exactly, so I tend to make changes. Sometimes my husband will rave about something I made and insist I write down the recipe. That's when I give him "the look," as he knows very well I never write anything down. I mentally make sure they are the healthiest possible recipes, although occasionally I splurge and prepare something a little less healthy. Like many people, I cook differently in the summer than the winter, fixing things we are in the mood to eat. It's not surprising that we prefer warm dishes when it's cold outside and opt for lighter fare like salads in the heat of summer.

Salads

Salads can surprise you. Most people believe they are eating healthfully when they head for the salad bar in restaurants, but that's not always the case. If you load your plate with cheeses, pasta and other starchy items, you may as well order a sandwich and actually consume far fewer calories. The salad dressings alone are usually extremely calorie-laden and may contain questionable ingredients. Making your own is a better way to go.

* **Black Olive Combo Salad:** Besides being tasty and colorful, this salad is good for you. Any of my salad dressings (*see Dressings section*) will work well here. A bonus: it will stay fresh in the fridge, with the dressing already mixed in, for at least three days. It's enough for 6-8 people, depending on what else is being served.

2 large cucumbers

4 Roma tomatoes

1 cup black olives

1 cup marinated artichoke hearts

1 medium sweet yellow onion

1 cup chopped red, yellow or orange peppers

Salt and pepper to taste

Chop the vegetables in small pieces and mix together in a bowl. Add enough salad dressing to completely cover all the ingredients, mixing well. Cover the bowl with aluminum foil or plastic wrap and chill until serving.

* **Broccoli Salad:** This salad will keep in the fridge for at least three days. It's a tasty way to get your daily dose of fiber and healthy broccoli. The crunchy

sunflower or pumpkin seeds add interest and lots of magnesium.

1 cup chopped broccoli

1 cup chopped cauliflower

1 cup chopped zucchini

1 cup chopped red onion

1 cup sunflower or pumpkin seeds

1 teaspoon each of tarragon and thyme

½ cup crumbled Feta cheese (optional)

Salt and pepper to taste

Steam the veggies for about 4 minutes, making sure they are still crisp and not mushy. Combine the veggies in a bowl and blend in the desired amount of salad dressing. Add the sunflower or pumpkin seeds.

* Marinated Cucumber Salad: A nice accompaniment to fish and seafood dinners, marinated cucumbers improve with age. This salad tastes better each day it is refrigerated and will stay fresh for at least four days.

2 large cucumbers

1 cup chopped green onions

¼ cup vinegar

1 teaspoon each of oregano, basil and thyme

Peel the cucumbers and slice very thin, setting them aside. Chop the onions and combine with vinegar and spices in a small bowl. Pour the vinegar/onion mixture over the cucumbers and blend well. Add salt and pepper to taste. Chill for at least three hours.

* **Celery Root Salad:** Every once in a while I bring home an ugly brown celery root to make one of my favorite salads. I have to admit I sneak in a little mayonnaise for good taste. The celery root takes some work peeling and cutting, but the taste is worth it. I first encountered this salad in France many years ago and have loved it ever since.

1 celery root

½ small onion

¼ cup yogurt

¼ cup mayonnaise

I teaspoon each of dill, oregano and thyme

Salt and pepper to taste

Peel the celery root and slice into very small sticks, or use a mandolin. Chop the onion very fine. Blend together the mayonnaise and yogurt, adding the spices, salt and pepper. Pour the dressing mixture into the salad and toss well.

* Tomato & Mozzarella Salad: For the best results, be sure to use only fresh, pre-sliced mozzarella and marinate the tomatoes.

6 Roma tomatoes, sliced lengthwise

1 lb. fresh mozzarella cheese, in ½ inch slices

fresh basil leaves, chopped

black olives

¼ cup olive oil

2 tablespoons wine vinegar

½ teaspoon each of basil, thyme, oregano and marjoram

Salt and pepper to taste

Blend the oil, vinegar and spices. Allow tomatoes to marinate for about an hour, then drain off excess. Line a plate with alternating slices of tomatoes and mozzarella. Season the salad with salt and pepper. Sprinkle chopped basil over all, and add a cup of black olives in the center of the plate.

* Mom's Best Coleslaw: This is an old family recipe my mother made. I plan ahead for this as it has quite a few ingredients. It sits well for days, if it's not devoured in one sitting! I make a lot of this tasty slaw to have for subsequent meals, or for just snacking.

1 head green cabbage

2 cups chopped cucumber

1 cup chopped red or yellow bell pepper

1 cup Feta OR blue cheese

½ cup chopped red onion

1 cup chopped green olives, pitted

½ cup peanuts

¼ cup olive oil

juice of one lemon

1 tablespoon oregano

1 teaspoon cayenne pepper

Slice the cabbage into very thin pieces about 1-inch long. Add the chopped veggies and the olives. Pour the olive oil and the lemon juice over the mixture. Add the seasonings and blend everything very well, salting to taste. Gently stir in the cheese. Add a large handful of fresh peanuts each time you serve.

* **Nutty Tuna Salad:** I enjoy this often for a quick

lunch. It is packed with vitamins and minerals and a healthy dose of omega 3. This makes enough to serve two.

1 small can Albacore tuna

2 tablespoons each of pumpkin seeds AND sunflower seeds

½ cup finely chopped celery

chopped romaine lettuce

¼ cup Greek yogurt

juice of one lemon

1 teaspoon each of dill weed, dry mustard and turmeric

Blend the tuna, seeds and celery well. Combine the yogurt, lemon juice and spices, add to the tuna and blend. Serve on a bed of chopped romaine. Salt and pepper to taste.

*Carrot, Celery & Pea Pod Salad: I generally purchase pea pods at the store when they are on sale, cooking up a batch with bean sprouts, mushrooms and other veggies. But I'm always sure to withhold a good portion of the pea pods to go into this favorite salad. They look especially festive with the orange color of the carrots.

1 cup pea pods

1 cup sliced carrots

1 cup sliced celery

1 8 oz. can water chestnuts

½ cup fresh, chopped parsley

For the dressing:

¼ cup sesame seed oil

¼ cup vinegar

2 tablespoons low-sodium soy sauce

1 teaspoon each of curry powder, garlic powder and lemon pepper spice

Cut the carrots and celery into thin slices. Remove the tough ends of the pea pods and cut in half. Add the water chestnuts and parsley and put all the ingredients into a bowl. Blend the dressing ingredients well. Toss the salad with the dressing and chill before serving.

* Chicken & Yogurt Salad: This is a delicious way to use leftover chicken. For a change of pace, you can warm this salad in the oven and have great results.

2 cups cooked chicken, cut in bite-size pieces

1 cup chopped celery

½ cup chopped green onions

½ cup each of flax seeds AND sesame seeds

1 cup plain yogurt

juice of one lemon

1 tablespoon each of turmeric, curry powder, fennel and garlic powder

salt and pepper to taste

Combine the chicken and vegetables. Blend the yogurt, lemon juice and spices, then pour over the chicken mix. Add the seeds and mix well. Add salt and pepper to taste. Chill the salad in the fridge for about two hours before serving. Alternatively, warm it in the oven at 200 degrees for 30 minutes.

* **Salmon Salad:** This is a great summertime lunch. It delivers our all-important dose of omega 3 along with lots of healthy veggies.

6 oz. can wild-caught salmon, drained

1 tablespoon mayonnaise

3 tablespoons yogurt OR sour cream

½ cup chopped celery

¼ cup sunflower seeds

1 squeeze lemon juice

1 teaspoon turmeric

1 teaspoon cumin

salt and pepper to taste

2 or 3 large spinach leaves

sliced fresh tomatoes

chopped green onions

Blend together the yogurt, mayonnaise and seasonings. Add the salmon, sesame seeds and celery, mixing together well. Serve on spinach leaves with the tomatoes and onions.

* **Purple Potato Salad:** These pretty little potatoes add a festive touch of color to a variety of dishes. Another bonus is their antioxidant power –it's four times as much as in an ordinary white potato. They do cost a bit more but I think they are well worth it. I enjoy making this potato salad as it feels healthy just using these ingredients, plus it tastes great! This recipe makes enough for six people, with some leftovers.

4 cups small purple potatoes

1 cup chopped bell peppers

1 cup chopped sweet onions

1 cup cooked turkey bacon

1 cup finely chopped celery

½ cup chopped parsley OR cilantro

½ cup chia seeds (optional)

For the dressing:

½ cup olive oil

¼ cup cider vinegar

1 tablespoon each of rosemary, turmeric and cumin

salt and pepper to taste

Boil the potatoes whole until they are done but still firm, and then cool to room temperature and chop into bite-sized pieces. Add the remaining veggies and the bacon to the potatoes. Mix together the dressing ingredients, then pour over the potatoes. Chill in the fridge, adding the chia seeds just before serving.

* Spinach & Feta Salad: Most of us were told when we were young to finish our vegetables, and spinach was usually the one we liked least. It's a sure bet that if Mom had fixed this salad we would have felt differently.

2 cups fresh spinach

2 green onions

½ cup finely chopped celery

5 chopped marinated artichoke hearts

½ cup pumpkin seeds

½ cup Feta cheese

Wash the spinach and green onions and dry with paper towel. Chop the spinach and green onion and add to bowl. Add the rest of the ingredients, one at a time. Cover with the salad dressing of your choice. (*see Dressing recipes)* Chill in fridge until serving.

* **Quinoa Salad:** Anytime I have leftover quinoa I fix this salad. Honestly, I often make a double recipe of quinoa just so I can. It makes a great main course when you're in the mood for something light.

2 cups cooked chicken breast, chopped

1 sweet red pepper, chopped

1 cup chopped walnuts

2 cups cooked quinoa

1 cup raw zucchini, chopped

1 teaspoon red pepper flakes

For the dressing:

1 cup Greek plain yogurt

juice of one lemon

I teaspoon each of rosemary, oregano and basil

Salt and pepper to taste

Blend the yogurt and spices. Pour the dressing over the chopped veggies, quinoa and chicken and mix thoroughly. Chill in the fridge for about an hour.

Salad dressings

I have been fixing my own salad dressings for as long as I can remember. I like knowing what goes into them, and since most commercial dressing labels read like a chemistry project I choose to make my own. The following recipes are simple and you can change or modify according to your personal tastes. I like my dressings very spicy and flavorful, but you may feel differently and choose to temper some of my suggestions.

I use mostly olive oil and avocado oil for the base, along with lemons and cider vinegar. You will also need a salad dressing bottle with a tight lid, a blender – this is optional but it certainly makes life easier -- and a whisk.

* Special Caesar Dressing

½ cup olive oil

¼ cup cider vinegar

2 tablespoons water

small tin of anchovies

1/4 cup grated Parmesan cheese (approx.)

1 teaspoon each of oregano, basil, thyme, tarragon and garlic powder

salt and pepper to taste

In a medium bowl, blend the olive oil, cider vinegar and water. Finely chop the anchovies and add to the oil mixture. Add all spices and salt and pepper, increasing the spices for a stronger tasting dressing. Add the Parmesan cheese and whisk until creamy and smooth. Transfer dressing into a container with a lid, in case there is some leftover for next time.

* **Mexican Dressing:** This one is easy. Simply blend all ingredients and enjoy!

½ cup avocado oil

¼ cup lemon juice

¼ cup water

1 tablespoon cumin powder

1 tablespoon oregano powder

½ teaspoon red pepper flakes

1 teaspoon garlic powder

salt and pepper to taste

* Italian Salad Dressing: Another easy one, just mix all the ingredients and whisk until smooth. Pour into salad dressing bottle for serving.

½ cup olive oil

¼ cup wine vinegar

¼ cup water

1 tablespoon each of oregano, basil and marjoram

½ teaspoon garlic powder

1 teaspoon fennel

salt and pepper to taste

* Dijon Salad Dressing: Blend all ingredients in a bowl and whisk briskly. Pour into lidded container and refrigerate.

½ cup grapeseed oil

¼ cup water

¼ cup cider vinegar

1 heaping tablespoon Dijon mustard

1 teaspoon each of thyme and rosemary

salt and pepper to taste

Soups

Once a month I cook up a large batch of black beans and white northern beans separately and then freeze them, dividing up the beans into quart containers. Doing this task in advance enables me to make soup in less than an hour. I just pull out the beans and let them defrost while I prepare the other soup ingredients. (I often make lentil soup but since lentils cook quickly I don't bother freezing them ahead of time.)

Very often I just use whatever I have on hand, and sometimes I buy special favorite veggies and healthful greens. Beans and veggies have a load of magnesium and I am committed getting enough of this vital mineral. To me it is a mainstay of good health. The amount of beans you put in your soup is up to you. I average about three cups per batch of soup, sometimes a bit more.

Despite their carefully measured ingredients, these recipes are very forgiving. You can add more or less veggies and seasonings, in fact, almost more or less of anything. Feel free to vary the amounts, as most proportions will usually work out deliciously.

My husband and I enjoy soup for lunch every day whenever we are at home. This saves us thinking about what to fix, and when I am away my husband can help himself to a healthy meal with little fuss. All of these soups freeze well.

* The Kitchen Sink: This soup will vary with what I happen to have in the fridge, and often incorporates vegetables I may have otherwise discarded. Over the years I have experimented with some really unusual veggies and the soup has always turned out great. I have used Brussels sprouts, red peppers, red cabbage, green onions, spinach and even radishes, something most people overlook when making soups. Go wild with this and you'll be delighted with your empty veggie bins.

large pot of water

2 tablespoons olive oil

2 tablespoons lemon juice

1 15 oz. can tomato sauce

salt and pepper to taste

Boil the water and add all the ingredients, including the veggies chopped in small pieces. I often toss in some crumbled cooked hamburger for a rich, meaty flavor, or some chicken and rice. Get creative with the spices and add your favorites.

* **Amazing Vegetable Stock:** I came across this idea online and found it to be one of the best ways to use all those veggies in the fridge that are on the wane.

large pot of water

2 tablespoons oil (olive, avocado or grapeseed)

2 1-gallon bags frozen veggie pieces

rosemary, thyme, ginger, curry powder and garlic powder to your taste

Put all your veggie leftovers from other recipes in a plastic bag and freeze. I usually wait to make this stock until I have two full bags. Boil the water with the seasonings, except the salt and pepper. Add the oil and simmer until all veggies are very tender, about two hours. Drain the soup and discard the veggies. Store the remaining liquid in containers and refrigerate or freeze until you need stock for any soup.

* **Tomato & Black Bean:**

3 cups cooked black beans

2 cups chopped tomatoes

1 large onion, diced

1 cup chopped cilantro

¼ cup avocado OR coconut oil

4 tablespoons each of cumin, oregano, basil and thyme

2 tablespoons red pepper flakes

juice of one lemon

Fill a large soup pot three-quarters with water, leaving room for all the ingredients. For an extra flavor boost, substitute chicken broth for some of the water. Add veggies and spices, except for the salt. Heat until boiling. Add the black beans and oil. Simmer for about 30 minutes, and then add salt and pepper to taste.

* White Beans & Garlic:

4 cups white beans, frozen or canned

1 quart water

1 quart vegetable stock, or more water

½ cup chopped parsley

1 cup chopped green onions

3 cups chopped fresh spinach

4 garlic cloves, chopped

2 tablespoons avocado OR olive oil

seasonings to your taste: rosemary, marjoram, thyme, salt and pepper

Thaw the beans, or drain thoroughly if you are using canned beans. Combine the water and vegetable stock and bring to a boil. Add the beans; they can be slightly frozen. Add the fresh veggies, the garlic and the oil. Add all seasonings except salt and pepper. Simmer for about 30 minutes, adding salt and pepper to taste.

* **Chicken & Brown Rice:**

4 boneless, skinless chicken thighs, chopped into bite-size pieces

2 cups raw brown rice

2 cups each of chopped celery, chopped sweet onions and chopped spinach

1 cup chopped zucchini

4 quarts water (or substitute one quart with chicken broth)

1 cup chopped parsley OR cilantro

2 tablespoons each of thyme, oregano, rosemary, marjoram, garlic powder and curry powder

1 teaspoon each of red pepper flakes and dried ginger

¼ cup grapeseed oil

salt and pepper to taste

Add water and chicken stock to a large pot over high heat. Add the rice and chicken and reduce heat to medium. Add the remaining vegetables and the seasonings, except for salt and pepper. Cook until the rice and veggies are tender. Add salt and pepper to taste. For a thicker soup, use less water. And for extra flavor, add any chicken or beef bones you may have, making sure to discard them before serving.

* **Chicken & Quinoa:** I try to include a lot of quinoa in my diet because its natural great taste is boosted with vitamins, minerals and amino acids. Quinoa is a seed so it is safe for those who are on gluten-free diets. This soup is a great way to warm up during cold weather. I make a lot of it and stock my freezer.

2 whole chicken breasts

4 quarts water

2 cups quinoa

1 cup chopped red onions

3 cups chopped kale

2 cups chopped bok choy

2 tablespoons each of oregano, basil, garlic powder and thyme

2 teaspoons each of turmeric and curry powder

¼ cup sesame OR olive oil

salt and pepper to taste

Add water to a large pot over high heat. Chop the chicken breasts into bite-sized pieces and set aside. Add kale to the water and cook for 15 minutes. Add all other veggies and spices. Add quinoa and simmer for about 30 minutes. Add the oil and chicken. Cook until the chicken is tender. Add salt and pepper to taste.

Vegetarian dishes

* **Cinnamon Carrots:** We've all heard the old saw that carrots are good for your eyesight. But did you also know they are also incredibly healthful for the entire body? I make this recipe about once a week as it is packed full of vitamins and minerals and one of my favorites, fresh turmeric root, to keep the brain sharp.

5 or 6 colorful carrots (yellow, red and white)

¼ cup olive oil

juice of one lemon

1 tablespoon each of ginger and cinnamon

4 tablespoons freshly grated turmeric root OR 2 tablespoons turmeric powder

salt and black pepper (Pepper is important as it actives the power of turmeric.)

Cut the ends off the carrots, and wash thoroughly. Steam the carrots until just tender but not mushy. Blend all ingredients except the salt in a small bowl. Pour the sauce over the cooked carrots, adding salt to your taste.

* Green Beans with Turmeric: We enjoy green beans often whenever they are in season. This particular recipe boasts added flavor from turmeric, making it doubly good for you. I'm always sure to make extra for munching on the next day.

fresh green beans (as much as you need)

¼ cup avocado oil

2 tablespoons cider vinegar

1 teaspoon each of oregano, fenugreek and basil

½ teaspoon red pepper flakes

2 tablespoons fresh grated turmeric

1 tablespoon black pepper

salt to taste

½ cup sunflower seeds

Steam the beans until tender. In a small bowl, blend all ingredients except the sunflower seeds. Pour mixture over the beans and toss, sprinkling the sunflower seeds over the top.

* Zucchini, Tomato & Onion Casserole: This luscious casserole will suffice for two meals, with a bit left for lunch. When zucchini is in season I prepare this fairly often.

3 cups thinly sliced zucchini

1 cup chopped onion

1 cup chopped tomatoes

½ cup chopped parsley

1 cup fresh Parmesan cheese

4 garlic cloves, chopped

¼ cup olive oil

juice of 1 lemon

2 tablespoons each of rosemary and oregano

salt and pepper to taste

In a small bowl, blend olive oil, lemon, garlic and all spices. Combine the veggies in a Pyrex baking dish, then add the oil mixture and toss thoroughly. Sprinkle the cheese over the vegetables, then bake at 350 degrees for about 1 hour.

* **Eggplant Casserole:** This healthy dish makes a great dinner when accompanied by a green salad. It lasts for two meals and then some, so it turns out to be quite economical. The layering of the veggies will vary with the size of your pan, so don't worry if you have the exact amount I show here. Sometimes I end up with only one layer, and it's always just as delicious!

1 medium eggplant

1 large sweet onion

6 or 7 Roma tomatoes, sliced

1 cup chopped celery

1 pound mozzarella cheese, grated or sliced thin

¼ cup olive oil

juice of 1 lemon

2 tablespoon each of oregano, basil, thyme and marjoram

1 teaspoon of cayenne pepper (optional)

salt and pepper to taste

Slice the eggplant into half-inch rounds. Salt the slices and score with a knife, then spread them on paper towels and let them sit for several hours. Mix the olive oil and spices, except for salt and pepper. Cover the bottom of a Pyrex baking dish with half of the olive oil mixture. Place a layer of eggplant on the bottom, then a layer of tomatoes followed by half of the onions. Add the celery. Cover the veggies with half the mozzarella cheese. Pour the remaining oil over the cheese. Add another layer each of eggplant, tomatoes and onions, ending with mozzarella cheese on top. Add salt and pepper to taste. Bake for about 1.5 hours at 350 degrees.

* Cheesy Cauliflower & Pumpkin Seeds: One of my weaknesses is cheese, so naturally this dish is high on my list of favorites. I never check the calories or fat because I don't want to know, as I consider this dish a real treat!

1 whole cauliflower

1 medium onion, diced

1 cup cheddar, provolone OR jack cheese, grated

pumpkin seeds (as many as you like)

1 tablespoon each of turmeric, curry powder, coriander and cumin

1 teaspoon red pepper flakes (optional)

salt and pepper to taste

¼ to ½ cup olive oil

Break the cauliflower into small flowerets, then cover with the oil and coat thoroughly. Add the onion and seasonings including salt and pepper and mix well. Pour the veggie mixture into an uncovered Pyrex baking dish. Top with the grated cheese of your choice and bake for 1 hour at 350 degrees.

* **Cabbage & Walnuts:** There's always a head of cabbage in my fridge, either red or white; they both work well for this recipe. This recipe pairs this very healthy vegetable with walnuts, another superfood brimming with omega 3. It makes a wonderful side to any main dish. And it tastes just as good the next day, if there's any left!

1 medium cabbage, chopped into medium pieces

1 small sweet onion, diced

1 cup chopped walnuts

¼ cup avocado oil

1 tablespoon each of thyme, basil and savory

salt and pepper to taste

water

Combine the seasonings. Heat the oil to high

temperature, and when it begins to sizzle add the seasonings and stir. Add the chopped cabbage and onions and stir, cooking over medium heat. After about five minutes, add ¼ cup of water to prevent the cabbage from sticking to the pan. Cover and simmer until it is cooked to your desired tenderness. Add the walnuts and simmer for one minute. Salt and pepper to taste.

A few favorite snacks

* Kale Chips

1 bunch kale

olive oil

lemon pepper spice

After removing the stalks, wash the leaves thoroughly and dry on paper towels. Cover the kale with 1 tablespoon of olive oil blended with the desired amount of lemon pepper spice. Spread the leaves on a non-stick cookie sheet, making sure they do not overlap. Bake at 350 degrees for about 20 minutes, or until the leaves are crispy.

* Baked Parmesan Crisps: I try not to make this treat too often, as it's always a struggle not to eat the entire batch before anyone else gets to it.

Grated fresh Parmesan cheese

Cover a cookie sheet with a layer of aluminum foil. Spread the grated Parmesan cheese thinly over the entire surface, making it as flat as possible. Sprinkle with black pepper. Bake in a pre-heated oven at 350 degrees until the cheese is brown and no longer bubbling. Turn off the oven, leaving the pan inside. The cheese will become a hard sheet. After about 15 minutes, remove the pan from the oven and carefully peel the cheese off the foil. Break into small serving pieces.

* **Baked Almonds:** I never buy pre-seasoned almonds because they usually contain far too much salt. Instead, I control the seasonings and happily accept the rave reviews.

1 pound almonds

olive OR avocado oil

1 tablespoon each of grated Parmesan cheese, black pepper and garlic powder

salt to taste

Mix the oil with the spices, pour the mixture over the almonds and coat them completely. Spread the almonds on a cookie sheet and bake at 350 degrees for about 30 minutes. Turn the oven off, letting the almonds sit for another half hour before removing from the oven.

* **No-Fail Hummus:** My habitual go-to appetizer when unexpected company stops by, this recipe is easy to prepare and healthful to eat. I generally cook beans from scratch, however I tried cooking raw garbanzo beans and was disappointed with the final result. So for this recipe I use the canned variety, opting for organic to minimize my guilt.

1 15-ounce can garbanzo beans, drained

¼ cup sesame seeds

juice of one lemon

2 tablespoons sesame seed oil

1 teaspoon each of curry powder, oregano and turmeric

salt and pepper to taste

Combine all the ingredients in a blender and pulse until totally smooth. Serve with crackers and celery stalks or other cut up veggies.

The main course

* **Pan-fried Fish with Nut Butter:** This dish looks and tastes just like what you would find on the menu in a seafood restaurant, except it is much better for

you. It's a perfect treat to make for the grandkids as they will surely love it and never dream they are eating something good for them!

2 cod filets per person

1 egg

½ cup milk (amount variable)

¼ cup EACH of finely chopped walnuts, sesame seeds, sunflower seeds, flax meal, pumpkin seeds and chia seeds. Or use any blend of these.

1 tablespoon each of dill, curry powder, turmeric, savory and coriander

1 teaspoon cayenne pepper (optional)

cooking oil: sesame seed, grapeseed OR avocado

salt and pepper to taste

Beat the egg with the milk. (You will need a second egg and more milk for more fish.) Combine the nut mixture with salt and pepper. Dip the filets on both sides in the egg mixture, then do the same in the nut mixture. Heat the oil in a large pan. Cook the filets, turning once, until the outside is crispy and the fish is tender and fully cooked.

* **Fish & Garlic Sauce:** This sauce works well for most types of fish that you might sauté. It is easy, healthful and delicious.

fish filets (the number depends on how many each person will eat)

5 cloves fresh garlic

2 tablespoons avocado oil

juice of one lemon

1 tablespoon EACH of tarragon, basil and thyme

pinch of cayenne pepper

salt and pepper to taste

Mince the garlic and add to the lemon juice in a small bowl. Add the avocado oil, spices, salt and pepper, blending well. Heat additional oil to cover the bottom of the pan. Add the filets to the pan and cover with the sauce. Turn the filets once. Cook the fish until it changes color and becomes opaque, then remove quickly from the pan and serve.

* Marinated Salmon & Capers: We love salmon and buy it whenever it is on sale. It's loaded with beneficial omega 3 and is really good for you, but actually we eat it because it's so delicious. It grills perfectly, but only if you have a perfect grill person on hand!

4 tablespoons olive oil

juice of one lemon

1 tablespoon Worcestershire sauce

¼ teaspoon red pepper flakes

1 teaspoon each of oregano and fenugreek

salt and pepper to taste

Combine all the ingredients. Pour the marinade over the salmon filets and put in the fridge. After about an hour, turn the filets and continue chilling until ready to cook. Grill the fish for as long as it takes to go from translucent to opaque, then remove from heat. Serve with lemon wedges and topped with 1 tablespoon of capers.

* Chicken with Artichoke Hearts & Mushrooms:
Most of us have favorite company dishes but this one is a surefire hit and healthy too. Besides, it's easy to make and never fails to please. Sometimes dinner isn't served at the exact time you plan and chicken breasts can become dry regardless of the sauce you've used. To avoid that, I use chicken thighs since they don't dry out despite extra cooking. This recipe will serve six, with two extra thighs for the big eaters. I use my large electric frying pan as I can control the heat more easily.

8 chicken thighs, with skin and bone

1 can non-marinated artichoke hearts

2 cups sliced fresh mushrooms

1 6 oz. can whole black olives

1 medium onion, chopped

grapeseed oil

2 tablespoons EACH of tarragon, basil and thyme

paprika, enough to cover thighs

1 cup dry white wine

Salt and pepper to taste

In a large frying pan, brown the chicken on both sides in the oil. Sprinkle with paprika and remove to a plate. Add more oil to the pan, then sauté the onion for five minutes. Add the seasonings to the mixture and return the thighs to the pan. Halve the artichokes and olives and add them to the chicken with the wine. Continue cooking over medium heat for about 15 minutes, or until the chicken is done. Taste the sauce, adding salt and pepper if desired. Turn off the heat for about ten minutes, then reheat before serving.

* **Chicken Veggie Mix:** Another version of my "kitchen sink" cooking technique, I gather almost every vegetable I can find in the fridge to make this quick, delicious baked chicken. If you're smart you'll prepare enough for at least two dinners, and be sure to include your favorite veggies.

chicken legs or thighs, on the bone, with skin (as many as you want)

2 tablespoons each of coconut oil OR sesame seed oil

¼ cup lemon juice

1 cup EACH of red sweet peppers, chopped onions, chopped spinach and chopped zucchini OR broccoli, cabbage, Brussels sprouts and tomatoes

2 tablespoons EACH of oregano, coriander, sage, fenugreek and basil

1 teaspoon cayenne pepper

salt and pepper

Preheat oven to 350 degrees. Blend the oil with the lemon juice, spices, salt and pepper. Rub this mixture over each piece of chicken. In a large baking dish, fit the veggies around the chicken. Add some salt and pepper to the veggies with a small amount of oil to cover them. Bake for about ninety minutes, or until the chicken is totally cooked.

* Spaghetti Squash & Ground Turkey: I love experimenting with recipes using this versatile vegetable that tastes almost like real spaghetti. Or close enough so that even picky eaters love it.

1 spaghetti squash

olive oil for rubbing

1 pound ground turkey

1 chopped onion

2 chopped tomatoes

1 can tomato sauce

3 garlic cloves, chopped

1 cup EACH chopped sweet red pepper and chopped cilantro

¼ cup avocado oil

2 tablespoons EACH of oregano, rosemary and coriander

paprika, salt and pepper to taste

Parmesan cheese

With a fork, poke holes around the squash, then rub well with olive oil. Bake for about one hour at 375 degrees until fork tender, then remove from the oven. Slice it lengthwise, discarding the seeds. Remove all the squash meat, by scraping with a fork and keep warm in a covered dish. Heat the avocado oil in a frying pan, add the garlic and brown the turkey. Add the remaining veggies and spices and cook over medium heat until turkey is done. (Add more oil if the turkey seems dry.) Pour in tomato sauce, adding salt and pepper to taste. Combine cooked turkey mixture with the spaghetti squash. Top off with Parmesan.

*** Vegetarian Spaghetti Squash:** About twice a month I make a purely vegetarian dinner. It helps me feel like I am saving the entire animal kingdom by not cooking meat. I typically serve this with a green salad and it lasts for two dinners and then some. After a day or two in the fridge it tastes even better and makes a great cold dish for lunch.

1 large spaghetti squash

2 cups chopped onions

2 cups sweet red peppers

½ cup chopped celery

1 cup chopped broccoli

4 garlic cloves, chopped

1 tablespoon EACH of ground fennel, oregano, dry mustard and ginger

avocado oil

salt and pepper to taste

¼ to ½ cup water OR vegetable broth

To cook the squash, follow the directions in the preceding recipe. While it's cooking, start the veggies.

Heat enough oil to cover the pan generously, then brown the garlic and remaining veggies. Blend the spices and add to the pan. Add water or broth. When veggies are tender but still crunchy, remove from heat and toss with the squash. Sprinkle generously with Parmesan.

Desserts

My husband and I rarely have desserts at home, although a few hours after dinner we may enjoy some fresh fruit. For dinner guests I usually set out a platter of cut-up fruit as most people have eaten enough and are no longer hungry. However I do have a favorite dessert for special occasions, and trust me, you cannot taste the avocados.

* Chocolate Avocado Mousse: This recipe will make enough for four small servings. It's rich and flavorful and yet still really healthful!

2 avocados

½ cup raw cocoa OR cacao powder

2-3 teaspoons xylitol (depending on your sweet tooth)

½ cup coconut OR almond milk

1 teaspoon liqueur: raspberry, mint or any flavor (optional)

Peel and chop the avocados into small pieces and add to a blender or bowl if using a hand mixer. Blend until smooth, then add the cocoa or cacao powder, sweetener and milk. Blend until mixture is smooth. Add in the liqueur and chill for at least two hours. For a festive touch, top with fresh raspberries, chopped nuts or shredded coconut.

*** Fresh Fruit Sauce:** Most of the time my husband and I eat our fresh fruit plain and love it that way. However, if you're craving a little something extra or are having guests for dinner, this sauce will surely bump it up a notch! You can use a variety of fruits such as berries, peaches, bananas, apricots or plums.

2 cups chopped fruit

1 cup Greek yogurt

1 tablespoon (or more) honey

5 strawberries

½ cup coconut

½ cup finely chopped walnuts

1 tablespoon rum (optional)

In a large bowl, blend the yogurt and honey. Finely chop the strawberries and add to the yogurt, along with the coconut and walnuts. Combine the chopped fruits with the yogurt mixture, then chill for another two hours before serving.

* Chocolate & Berries Fro-Yo: Although I love fruit in its natural state, once in a while I admit to craving something creamy and slightly sinful. This recipe is easy and will satisfy the most insistent sweet tooth!

2 cups frozen raspberries or strawberries (unsweetened)

2 tablespoons honey

1/3 cup plain full-fat yogurt

½ cup cocoa OR cacao powder

2 teaspoons rum extract (optional)

Combine all the ingredients in a blender and pulse until smooth, or with some small pieces of fruit remaining. Place the mixture in a plastic container and freeze for at least three hours. When completely frozen, remove from freezer and hand mix until creamy. Return the yogurt to the freezer for about one hour.

* Frozen Bananas: You'll be singing my praises after trying this fabulous dessert. It's one quick and delicious way to get your daily dose of potassium!

3 bananas

1 tablespoon honey

2 tablespoons milk

3 tablespoons dark chocolate chips

Peel and freeze the bananas overnight. When they are frozen, place in blender with the honey and milk and pulse until smooth. Freeze the mixture in a plastic container until it is solid. Remove from freezer, add the chocolate chips and stir until creamy, then return to the freezer for about two hours.

Chapter 4: Homemade Health and Beauty

Making my own skin blends is surely fun, but an added bonus comes from knowing that using preservative-free ingredients is doing my body a great service. Using natural products on your skin will keep your entire body healthier and keep your immune system functioning at its peak.

Periodically I designate a "cooking day" and make all of my favorite products, which usually means I fix the easiest recipes that will produce the best results. You'll see that after you have gathered all the ingredients, these recipes pull together pretty quickly. Small glass Mason jars such as those used for canning jams and jellies are perfect for storing your finished products. Now get started on your own journey into personalized skin care!

Carrier oils

These are the oils that are blended with essential oils to dilute their strength and also make them easier to apply. Each one has its own special properties, and all of them offer nourishment to the skin and the entire body. Some oils are also suitable for cooking, and many work well for blending your own beauty products.

* **Coconut:** This oil has become very popular over the past several years, with many promises of various cures and health benefits. I use it for sautéing meats and veggies as it can reach high temperatures without smoking. Filled with natural antioxidants, it can be used on the hands, face and hair. Another of its advantages is that it naturally solidifies at room temperature, thus creating a sturdier base for blends. Sometimes when I am in the kitchen I'll reach for a dab or two and moisturize my hands and face.

***Sweet Almond:** As well as being suitable for cooking, sweet almond oil is rich in vitamin E and thus very soothing to the skin. It is moisturizing and nourishing, balancing the skin's natural oils.

* **Apricot Kernel:** This is one of my favorites: A great fighter against dry and irritated skin, it is particularly nourishing and thus good for facial and body creams. The oil is also suitable for cooking.

***Sesame:** My husband and I often use sesame oil in our cooking, especially in many of our favorite Asian dishes. The oil has a heavy density, is very flavorful, and can reach high temperatures without undergoing molecular changes. One of its many health benefits is richness in vitamins E and B complex. However, be aware that it has a fairly strong aroma and although it is compatible with other essential oils and very nourishing in foods, you have to really like the aroma!

*Olive: Certainly everyone is familiar with olive oil. It is a staple in my kitchen for just about everything, and probably yours too. This oil is light and works well for different health and beauty blends due to its moisturizing quality and nourishing content. It is best not used for cooking at high temperatures as it has a low smoking point. You may have heard something in the news about "fake" olive oil. To avoid running into this problem I buy Costco's own organic, cold-pressed, extra virgin oil, as it is certified pure.

* Jojoba: I reach for the bottle of jojoba oil I keep in the bathroom for a variety of uses. One way is directly out of the bottle when my skin feels very dry. Living as I do in a dry climate, I moisturize my face at least three times each day. An excellent carrier oil, jojoba mixes well with just about every other essential oil. This allows me to add a little of it to many different recipes. An extra bonus is its very long shelf life.

*Flaxseed: Flax meal has been lauded for many years as a great source of Omega 3, as well as other vitamins and minerals. Flaxseed oil is also popular for cooking and makes a great choice as a carrier oil due to its anti-inflammatory properties.

* Pomegranate: Known for its healing properties, pomegranate oil is used for both cooking and skin care. It is anti-inflammatory and also a strong antioxidant, making pomegranate an outstanding choice for a carrier oil.

* **Avocado:** Many people think of avocados as a vegetable, but it is actually a fruit. Popular in salads, as a major part of guacamole, in sandwiches and sauces, delicious avocados are filled with fiber, minerals and vitamins. The oil is touted to be extra-nourishing for aging skin. So whether you cook with it or use it for your carrier oil, it is tops. I use this oil a lot for sautéing vegetables because of its mild flavor and high smoking point.

Recipes for a healthier you

* **Lip Balm or Gloss:** This recipe allows you to substitute different butters, such as mango butter. You can purchase empty tubes for filling with your own balm that are just like the commercially prepared products you find in stores. However, I find it easier to use small glass jars and simply apply the balm with my fingertips.

Chocolate Mint Lip Balm
What could be bad about combining chocolate and mint? I love this flavor; using it makes me feel like I'm having a special treat.

1 tablespoon cocoa butter
1 tablespoon plus 1 teaspoon beeswax pellets
2.5 tablespoons sweet almond oil OR apricot kernel oil
1 tablespoon avocado oil

2 to 3 drops Vitamin E oil
10 drops peppermint essential oil

Combine cocoa butter, beeswax, almond oil and avocado oil in a Pyrex measuring cup. Place it in a larger pan filled with about 2 inches of water. Cook over a medium flame until the mixture is smooth and everything is melted. Add the vitamin E oil and 20 drops of peppermint essential oil.
Pour the mixture into glass containers, leaving the lids off until it is completely cool. Optional: Use Shea butter instead of cocoa and add lavender essential oil.

* **Peppermint Toothpaste:** Making my own toothpaste allows me to avoid unhealthy additives like sugar, preservatives and other mystery ingredients found in most commercial brands. I like to prepare it in small batches fairly often and change the flavor, using lemon essential oils, lavender or wintergreen. After much prodding I convinced my husband to try it, and now he uses it exclusively!

½ cup coconut oil
2-3 tablespoons baking soda
15-20 drops peppermint, or essential oil of your choice

Blend the coconut oil and baking soda until smooth, then add the peppermint oil and blend. Transfer mixture to a glass container and place in the fridge to set. When it is thick but spreadable and slightly grainy, it's ready. For super-cleaning, add half a teaspoon of Himalayan salt. For a sweeter taste, add a teaspoon of xylitol, a sweetener that supports healthy gums and teeth.

* **Sunscreen:** Lately there's been a lot of negative buzz about how using commercial sunscreens may be responsible for bad skin conditions. To stay safe, here is my guaranteed healthful recipe for sunscreen you can use with confidence whenever you spend time outdoors.

All the oils used here have some SPF, but carrot seed oil and pomegranate seed oil are both very high. You can add different amounts of zinc oxide to the blend depending on how much skin protection you wish. Two tablespoons of zinc oxide equals 15 SPF. Besides having a high SPF, zinc oxide benefits your skin in other ways: It improves wound healing, treats acne and keeps the skin moist.

¾ cup coconut oil
1 tablespoon pomegranate oil OR carrot seed oil
2 tablespoons of Shea butter, which has a high SPF
2-4 tablespoons zinc oxide
2-6 drops of essential oil
Optional oils for fragrance (Do not use citrus oils as they have a negative reaction in sunlight.)

Combine the first three ingredients in a Pyrex cup and set in a pan filled with two inches of water. Place over medium heat. Heat and stir often until everything is melted, then remove from the stove. Add the zinc oxide and essential oils and blend well, then store in cool place. If the mixture is too thick, leave it out on the counter for a few hours before adding about 1 teaspoon of either sweet almond oil or apricot kernel oil, and mix in thoroughly. These oils never harden, unlike coconut oil.

* **Skin Exfoliator:** I love this simple recipe for sugar scrub as it has only three ingredients. I exfoliate with it about once a week. It is probably the only time I use sugar!

½ cup coconut oil
2 cups white sugar
12-15 drops of any essential oil (I like rosemary, lavender and lemon grass.)

Blend all the ingredients. If the mixture is too hard, add another teaspoon of carrier oil. Refrigerate for at least one hour before using.

***Brown Sugar Scrub:** Blend the ingredients in a small bowl, then transfer to a glass container and refrigerate for a few hours.

1/4 cup brown sugar
2 tablespoons olive or avocado oil
1 tablespoon cocoa powder

* **Body Cream:** Aloe vera gel has a well-deserved reputation as a skin soother. This particular recipe is quick and easy with no cooking involved. I have made it using a blender but have found that mixing by hand works just as well. I apply this cream after a shower and before I go to bed.

1.5 cups coconut oil
4 teaspoons aloe vera gel
1 teaspoon rosehips seed essential oil
12-15 drops lavender, Frankincense or sweet orange essential oil

Whisk together the first two ingredients. Pour this mixture into a bowl and refrigerate for about an hour. Add the essential oils and blend well, then store into glass jars with lids.

* **Facial Moisturizer:** This produces an amazing facial moisturizer using just two ingredients. I love jojoba oil as it resembles the skin's natural oil. Sometimes when I'm in a hurry I just pour a little of it onto my hands and massage my face.

1 teaspoon jojoba oil
1 teaspoon Frankincense oil

Blend these two ingredients together. For variety, add a few drops of lavender essential oil. Love that lavender! For a different twist, try this recipe for a facial moisturizer that doesn't use coconut oil.

½ cup Shea butter
¼ cup of either jojoba, sweet almond or apricot kernel oil (you can add coconut oil if you wish at this point)
3 drops carrot seed oil
5 drops of either rosemary, geranium or lavender essential oils

Combine the butter and other chosen oil in a Pyrex cup and set in a pan in 2 inches of water. Melt over medium heat until blended. Transfer to a glass bowl and chill thoroughly. Add the essential oils, mixing everything well. Store in small glass jars with lids.

* **Facial Cleanser:** I love how clean and smooth this non-soap cleanser leaves my skin feeling, so I use it twice a day. This blend goes together fast, so I can make a new batch even when I'm short on time. Simply combine all ingredients and pour into glass jars.

1 cup coconut oil
1 tablespoon baking soda
5 drops EACH of lavender essential oil, Frankincense essential oil and lemon essential oil

* **Shampoo and Body Wash:** This is my favorite shampoo and body wash combo. Besides being quick to make, the ingredients are pure, without any of the toxic additives found in most commercial brands. My very unruly hair has turned gray, so I color it about every six weeks. It's no surprise that after years of bleach, my hair is dry and wild at times. This shampoo is so gentle, I am once again enjoying a happy relationship with my hair.

½ cup Castile soap
½ cup pure water
6 drops rosemary essential oil
1 tablespoon baking soda

Blend all ingredients well in a Pyrex cup and pour into a clean and sterilized pump bottle. That's it!

Body Butter: Frequent applications of body butter offer another way to stave off the dry skin that seems to come with age. Living in a very dry climate, I use it several times a day. You can keep things interesting by trying a variety of essential oils.

1 cup organic raw Shea butter
½ cup coconut oil
½ cup of either almond or apricot kernel oil
10 drops of essential oils: lavender, lemon, rose or geranium

Melt the Shea butter and coconut oil in a Pyrex cup set inside a large pot with about two inches of boiling water. Cool the mixture until it begins to solidify, then whip with a hand whisk. Cool until smooth and melted. Add the almond or apricot oil along with additional essential oils of your choice.

* **Energy Mix:** I like to think that I have just as much energy as I did when I was younger, but that it just doesn't last as long. For those times when I am feeling tired and have something I have to do or somewhere I have to be, this works wonders. I simply dab a little behind my ears and wrists; besides the pleasant scent, it's a sure pick-me-up.

As always, use a carrier oil to dilute the essential oils. As a general rule, one tablespoon of essential oils requires about 10 tablespoons of coconut oil. I use mostly coconut oil for my blends as it results in a more solidified end product. Use this mixture sparingly and it will last you a very long time.

6 drops lemon essential oil
4 drops peppermint essential oil
8-10 drops rosemary essential oil or basil essential oil
¼ cup coconut oil
1 tablespoon sweet almond oil

Blend all ingredients well and chill for about an hour. Store in a small glass container.

* **Foot Cream:** After a long day on my feet I eagerly indulge myself with this cream, applying it right after a cleansing shower. My feet feel great and I feel relaxed.

½ cup coconut oil

1 tablespoon apricot kernel oil
4 drops each: peppermint essential oil, rosemary essential oil, lavender essential oil, clary sage essential oil

Combine all ingredients and blend well, then pour mixture into a glass container and refrigerate it until it is solid. If the mixture is too thick and hard to use, warm it in the microwave and add an additional teaspoon of apricot kernel oil, again blending well.

* **Rice Water Foot Soak:** This unusual recipe for a foot soak uses rice water, which is said to be beneficial for the circulation.

½ cup rice
2 to 3 cups rice water
2 tablespoons baking soda
10 drops of essential oil, either tea tree or lavender

Simmer half a cup of rice in 4 quarts of water until rice is cooked through. There should be about 2 cups of rice water left over. Pour the remaining water into a large bowl. Add enough warm water to the bowl to cover your feet. Blend in the baking soda and add the essential oils. Soak your feet while the liquid is still warm, and follow with a foot massage using the preceding cream blend.

* **Easy Foot Soak:** Another quick fix for tired feet, simply blend the warm water and salt, then add the

essential oils. Soak feet until the water starts to cool. Dry your feet and massage with the foot cream blend.

2 quarts warm water
½ cup sea salt
4 drops each of your choice of essential oils: peppermint, lavender, eucalyptus or lemon

* **Sore Muscle Salve:** My memory may not be what it once was, but I don't remember experiencing so many aches and pains when I was younger, unless I strained a muscle or ran a half-marathon. Now it's not so rare around our house. My husband was complaining about sore muscles after we rode our bikes the other day, so I whipped up this brew and he felt better soon after using it. Or at least he stopped complaining!

½ cup coconut oil
½ cup apricot kernel oil
5 drops each of these essential oils: ginger, thyme, cypress, marjoram and rosemary

Blend both the oils together with the essential oils until smooth. Chill in the fridge for about an hour. Here's another quick recipe for aches and pains; combine the ingredients and store in a glass container:

10 drops peppermint oil
2 tablespoons coconut oil

Stress Mix: Since stress is part of everyday life, ease it with this soothing blend and add some calmness to your day. Of course the problems will not disappear but your attitude will improve and help you cope. A therapist may help us to get to the root of our problems, but this stress blend can help alleviate some of our immediate negative feelings.

6 drops lavender oil
6 drops rose oil
6 drops bergamot essential oil
¼ cup coconut oil
1 teaspoon apricot kernel oil

Blend all ingredients until smooth, and then chill in the fridge for an hour or two. If the blend is too solid, add a few drops of the apricot kernel oil and let it sit on the counter. Cautionary Note: Using essential oils during pregnancy may be risky for some women. This may not apply to you but perhaps you will be making some of my products for a young friend or family member. I strongly recommend checking with your health provider before using any essential oils during pregnancy.

Chapter 5: Household Cleaning Solutions

When we were younger, it seemed like we could handle toxic environments more easily. We hardly noticed being in smoke-filled rooms, eating too much sugar, getting sufficient sleep and just being careless about our health. Young people think they are immortal, taking many chances in life that we don't later on in life. Either we get smarter or just become more cautious; either way, it's not unusual to make healthier decisions as we age.

The flip side is that as we age, our bodies become less forgiving. Regardless of our smart health practices, wise food choices, and attention to exercise, we still have to take extra pains to stay vigorous. Keeping our homes free from toxins as much as we can will go a long way towards keeping us healthy as we age. What better way to do this than using natural products? And though we can't control all the toxicity present in the environment, we can certainly lessen it in our homes with our homemade products.

Since I dislike the fumes that result from aerosol cans and the mixing of different fragrances from various store-bought cleaners, I use only natural ingredients in my household cleaners. At first it may seem like a lot of work, but actually all of these cleaners come together quickly and require only a few ingredients to produce. The first step is purchasing a few spray bottles and some labels to keep them separate. The rest is easy.

Although I use these recipes for general cleaning, sometimes I just grab a trusty clean rag and dip it in bowl of baking soda and give the kitchen sink, counter tops and bathrooms a once-over, making sure to rinse everything with warm water as the baking soda leaves a residue. I am confident that the baking soda leaves everything clean and sanitized.

White vinegar is a great choice for many cleaning solutions, but it does have a very strong smell that will dissipate after about an hour. I have read that white vinegar does not do well on granite and tile, but so far I haven't had a problem. It's your call, and I do offer some substitutes.

* **Easy Kitchen Cleaner:** Combine the following ingredients in a spray bottle to produce a quick, multi-purpose cleaning solution.

1 cup distilled vinegar
2 cups water
5 drops favorite essential oil: lemon, lavender or grapefruit

***Baking Soda Cleaner:** Blend all ingredients in a small bowl, adding the baking soda slowly as it tends to drift away. Then simply pour the mixture into a spray bottle and get busy!

1 cup water
1 cup white vinegar
3 tablespoons baking soda
5-6 drops essential oil

* **Borax Cleaner:** Blend the following ingredients and pour mixture into a pump bottle.

1 teaspoon borax
2 tablespoons Castile soap
½ teaspoon washing soda (See recipe below.)
6-7 drops of essential oil: lemon, geranium, lavender or rose
2 cups water

* **Washing Soda:** One day when I was at home and had some free time, I got ambitious and did some experimenting with this recipe. Since then I have made it frequently and am constantly amazed by its cleaning ability. The baking process strengthens the power of the baking soda. Adding one cup of water will produce a thin paste. You can also use it without adding any water, or add even more water to use it in a spray bottle. Be sure to watch the time and remember you have baking soda cooking -- the first time I did this I ended up with very dark baking soda!

2 cups baking soda
large cookie sheet

Preheat oven to 400 degrees. Spread the baking soda over the cookie sheet and bake for one hour. Remove the pan from the oven and smooth out the soda with a spatula. Bake another hour, then remove from oven and transfer soda to a plastic container. Optional: Add one cup of water, blending well.

* **Wood Cleaner:** We all know that wooden cabinets in the kitchen can get greasy and grimy. I use this cleaner about once a week and enjoy its lemon scent. Before using this mixture on your wood, try a sample to ensure it doesn't harm the wood.

1 cup water
¾ cup white vinegar
3 tablespoons olive oil
6 drops of lemon or sweet orange essential oil

Mix all ingredients and transfer to a spray bottle. Shake gently before using.
* **Windows and Mirrors:** This mixture is so simple to make, and naturally non-toxic. I am more apt to clean my mirrors when the supplies are handy, so I keep one spray bottle in each bathroom, with a clean rag. Every so often I will give my windows the once-over with this mixture. Mix all ingredients in a spray bottle, and use with a clean rag or a sponge.

¼ cup white vinegar
1 cup water
juice of half a lemon

If you have some rubbing alcohol on hand, here's another one to try for cleaning your glass and mirrors. Blend ingredients in a spray bottle, then spray and wipe with a microfiber rag. Adding a few drops of lemon essential oil will lend a pleasant scent.

1 cup water
1 cup rubbing alcohol
1 tablespoon white vinegar

* Disinfectant Spray: With pets in the house -- we have cats -- I use this spray often, and they don't seem to mind the pleasant scent. I also spray this directly onto the furniture and it keeps everything fresh. Make sure to pre-test your fabric furniture for colorfastness. Gently combine the ingredients to keep the baking soda from drifting. Pour mixture into a spray bottle and use liberally to disinfect, especially when someone in the house is sick.

½ cup baking soda
2 tablespoons Castile soap
1 teaspoon hydrogen peroxide
1-2 cups water, depending on the size of the spray bottle

* Kitchen Hand Soap: For years, after I finished cleaning up in the kitchen, I always reached for the dish detergent. No more; now I use this mixture instead and find it to be much gentler on my hands.

Blend all ingredients and mix well, then add to a pump bottle and keep it handy. You will marvel at how soft your hands feel after using this soap.

1 cup Castile soap
¼ cup water
5 to 6 drops of essential oil (Use your favorite; I prefer lemon or lavender.)

* Drain Cleaner: One day my husband noticed a bad odor in the kitchen. Following his nose, he discovered it was coming from the garbage disposal. Soon after, I used this cleaner and it worked wonders; the next time he entered the kitchen he said nothing, always a good sign! The lemony scent is a bonus, particularly after using the garbage disposal. I keep this handy in the kitchen so I'll remember to spray the drain every few days.

2 tablespoons grated lemon zest
1 tablespoon baking soda
1 cup water

Simply grate the lemon peel, then add it to the water and baking soda in a spray bottle. Shake gently.

* Carpet Stain Remover: Commercial carpet stain remover may do the job but also may leave an unpleasant odor. Both of the following recipes avoid that and work just as well. The first one uses baking soda and is good for pet stains and removal of pet odors. It is advisable to test a small area of your carpet first to be sure it is colorfast to the vinegar.

baking soda
white vinegar
Shake a generous amount of baking soda onto the stain and let it set for about an hour. Pour white vinegar on the baking soda and it will start to fizz. Rub the stain with a dry rag and allow it to dry. Finally, vacuum the area.

Here's one to try that uses common table salt and also works well on fabric:

table salt
white vinegar
water

Sprinkle a generous amount of salt on the stain and let is set for about 45 minutes. Combine one part white vinegar with two parts warm water in a spray bottle. Spray mixture over the salted area. When completely dry, vacuum.

* **Bathroom Scrub:** When it's time to seriously scrub down the bathrooms, I use this mixture. It really leaves everything sparkling. Blend the ingredients and store in a glass jar or container. Simply pour the mixture onto the sink, toilet and tub and let it sit for about an hour, then scrub with a damp, microfiber

rag. Rinse with warm water to avoid leaving any residue.

Some people claim that salt may scratch a fiberglass finish, but so far I haven't noticed any problems.

1 cup borax
1 cup baking soda
½ cup sea salt

* **Natural Bleach:** This is a great substitute for commercial bleaches. Store this mixture in a covered jar until ready to use, and then pour a small amount onto floors or countertops. Finish off with a rag soaked in warm water.

1 cup baking soda
1 tablespoon Castile soap
½ teaspoon hydrogen peroxide

* **Cutting Board Cleaner:** Because cutting boards absorb a lot of bacteria, I clean mine every day before use. This is a simple and easy fix: Just slice a lemon in half and rub it over the board and you're good to go!

* **Granite Cleaner:** Having heard from several sources that white vinegar was not advisable for granite countertops I devised this simple recipe. Blend ingredients in a spray bottle and make sure to put a label on it.

½ cup rubbing alcohol

1 teaspoon dish detergent
2 cups warm water

Chapter 6: A Wellness-Stocked Cupboard

The products that I use most often for cooking, cleaning and mixing up my many creams and potions offer many benefits. Better health and a cleaner, non-toxic home environment can be in your future as well if you keep these products on hand, as I have for years.

* Baking Soda: For a variety of uses, I reach for baking soda just about every day. Besides being an ingredient in my household cleaning recipes and my toothpaste, baking soda deodorizes and disinfects. It's also the quickest and easiest remedy for heartburn: Simply mix a teaspoonful in a glass of water and drink it down. Not great tasting but your heartburn disappears, and it's better than taking a drug.

Baking soda makes a great soak for tired feet. For a natural deodorant, rub a little under your arms and brush off the excess. I keep a small box of baking soda open inside the fridge to absorb food odors, and always have another large one on hand for emergency cleanups and whatever else comes along.

* Lemons and Lemon Peels: Because of their great scent and pungent taste, I add some lemon to almost everything I cook. They are loaded with vitamin C and antioxidants, are anti-inflammatory and have proven cardiovascular benefits. The true hero of the lemon is the peel. It's loaded with vitamins and minerals and adds a surprising amount of flavor to foods. It's a good idea to buy organic lemons since many times you will be eating the skin.

The best way to use the peel is to first wash a few lemons thoroughly, then put them in a plastic bag and place in the freezer. Freezing makes it easier to grate the peel later on when you are using it in cooking.

Since I drink a lot of water throughout the day, I generally add a splash of lemon juice and a tiny bit of xylitol for some quick healthy lemonade. So I guess you could say that when life gives me lemons, I make lemonade!

* **Cacao Powder:** While most people are familiar with cocoa powder, far fewer know its healthier counterpart, *cacao* powder. The two may be close in spelling but have far different properties. Cacao power is cocoa in its natural state, before any refining or heat treatment, and contains about four times the antioxidant power of dark chocolate. And really, who doesn't love chocolate?

Cacao powder can improve heart health, lower stress levels and decrease inflammation. I put a teaspoon in my morning coffee and may add it to different soups and casseroles during the day. My delicious *Avocado Mousse*, which can be found in the recipe section of this book, uses cacao powder. In fact, whenever any recipe you run across calls for cocoa powder, you might try substituting this superior version instead.

* Cider Vinegar: The health claims of this vinegar are broad, with many people believing that it cures just about anything. While all vinegars, whether white, red, or cider, actually do kill many types of bacteria, I still believe there's no magic bullet that can cure everything. Health benefits aside, I always stock a bottle of cider vinegar in my pantry for use in for salad dressings and adding to homemade soups. Vinegar adds lots of flavor and cuts back on salt use, another potential health benefit.

*Hydrogen Peroxide: Like many teenagers did years ago before the crazy hair colors of today's youth, I experimented with hydrogen peroxide to bleach my hair, applying it with cotton balls and then sitting in the sun until I achieved a lovely red/orange color. These days I often add a few drops to my toothpaste recipe for extra whitening power. Whatever your goal, be sure to use only 3% hydrogen peroxide solution for any personal uses.

It's wise to keep a separate spray bottle for a hydrogen peroxide mixture, which is one part hydrogen peroxide to four parts water. If you are plagued with mold in your house, use this spray and let it sit for about an hour, then happily see it disappear.

I also use it to wash fruits and vegetables, soaking them for about 30 minutes and then rinsing thoroughly with water. The solution is also effective for removing red wine stains, and in fact works well for just about any type of cleaning task. Although I haven't yet tried this personally, I've been told that if you leave some on your fingernails for about an hour it will whiten them.

* **Xylitol:** This is my go-to sweetener. I like it because it is 100% natural and tastes good, with the additional perk of containing 40% fewer calories than sugar. Of course it's healthier for your teeth and gums, and also helps regulate your blood sugar. Approved by the FDA for use in a variety of commercial products, you use the same amount of xylitol as sugar for sweetening power. For those of you who add sugar or artificial sweeteners in your coffee or tea, this is the healthful way to go.

***Chia Seeds:** These little black seeds pack a wallop with their healthy minerals, vitamins, dietary fiber, protein and omega-3. I keep them on hand and add them to soups, salads, meatloaf and casseroles. Two tablespoons of chia seeds provide 30% of your daily magnesium requirement. They are naturally low in calories and can be eaten whole.

* **Flaxseeds:** Whether you use them whole, ground or in oil, flaxseeds are a must-have in every health-conscious home. This superfood is a great source of soluble fiber, protein and alpha-linoleic acid, an omega-3 fatty acid. Mix flaxseeds into your morning smoothie and lunchtime yogurt, or sprinkle them

generously over a dinner salad. But remember to always drink a big glass of water when eating the seeds, or you run the risk of constipation.

I stock both the seeds and the meal for use in different recipes. Flax meal is great in meatloaf in place of oatmeal or breadcrumbs. Cold-pressed flaxseed oil should never be heated and only used for cold dishes. It's best to store it in the refrigerator.

Raw Nuts: Almonds, walnuts, pistachios and cashews are always ready for healthy snacking. Munching on nuts keeps you from reaching for empty calories in sugary snacks or other processed food. Though they are high in calories they are also high in vitamins, minerals and omega-3. Just a handful is filling and gives a burst of protein-fueled energy. They are best unsalted, although I occasionally I will bake the nuts with a variety of seasonings as a special treat or as holiday gifts. They will stay fresh for a long time when stored in an airtight container.

Legumes: The best part about always having legumes in your pantry is their ready availability and lack of an expiration date. If and when I run out of perishable foods, I can always count on beans or lentils to supply a healthy side dish. Legumes are filled with vitamins and minerals and also help regulate your blood sugar. They offer another way to get the magnesium you desperately need, as well as the fiber. I usually purchase fresh beans that require soaking before using, but I do keep a few cans of organic black, white and garbanzo beans in the pantry for last-minute meals. I generally buy organic and always drain and rinse the beans.

* **Castor Oil:** Castor oil has been around for hundreds of years and was often used as a cure-all for a great many conditions. Known to boost circulation, fight skin infections and help heal wounds, it's also a boon for muscle soreness. Just mix castor oil with lemon grass essential oil and apply to the painful area. After about ten minutes you'll get sweet relief!

I do not recommend using this oil internally, as there are still many pros and cons concerning this. However, there are plenty of external uses for this amazing oil. Since my home state of Arizona has a very dry climate, I tried mixing the castor oil with coconut oil with great results: after one application, I found that my skin didn't need to be rehydrated all day long. That's quite a change from the commercial creams I had been slathering on three or four times a day.

***Black, White and Green Tea:** Besides enjoying it for its flavor, there is literally a type of tea for everything that ails you. You can find teas to treat upset stomachs, colds, headaches, painful joints, and more. There are teas with hibiscus for controlling high blood pressure, ginger or fennel for soothing an upset stomach, and eucalyptus for clearing up congestion.

Truthfully, you could devote a whole shelf in your pantry for all the varieties available.

Of course you can go for black, green or white, and the lesser-known varieties like oolong and pu-erh. We've all heard for years about the benefits of green tea, however to ignore the other two cousins -- white and black --might be foolish. I keep some specialty teas in the house in case we have a last minute need.
Whatever you choose, it's important to know that the less processed the tea, the healthier it is for you.

Made of steamed leaves, green tea is alleged to interfere with a variety of different cancers and support the body's neurological functions. It may also lower cholesterol levels. Black tea is made with fermented leaves and has the highest caffeine content. It offers protection of the cardiovascular system. White tea is uncured and unfermented; one study showed it to have potent anti-cancer properties.

* **Aloe Vera:** Available in liquid, cream and gel, aloe vera is gentle on the skin and thus is often used for treating sores, bug bites and rashes. Because of that I have incorporated aloe vera gel into some of my most soothing skin creams. Those suffering with stomach issues will benefit from a dose of aloe vera juice. It is said to protect your immune system and be healthy for the heart. However, before taking it internally check with your health provider to ensure it won't cause problems with any prescription drugs you may

take or health conditions you may have.

*Himalayan Salt: Salt is an important part of a healthy diet, as long as you don't overdo it. It regulates the water content throughout your body and regulates blood sugar levels. Himalayan salt is the only kind I use, being surprisingly low in sodium and 100% pure. Best of all, I avoid feeling guilty about using salt; full of healthy minerals, it is far superior to table salt.

* Vitamin C Powder: There are so many benefits from this vitamin for your skin, teeth, immune system and nervous system. (For more on the importance of vitamin C in our diets, see Chapter 2.) As most of us are aware, today we may get fewer vitamins and minerals from our food due to soil deficiency. To compensate, I keep a jar of this powder handy and add some to my daily water. Particularly when the cold and flu season hits, I never miss my daily dose.

* Brown Rice: Some meals just call for rice. My husband and I enjoy having shrimp for dinner every few weeks, and rice is a must. I prefer the brown, long-grain organic rice available at Costco. Brown rice has a shorter shelf life than white, lasting about six months. But it's rich in vitamins and minerals with the sheath left on the rice, and also contains a healthy amount of magnesium. I make mine in a rice cooker because cooking rice in high altitudes seems to take forever. However you make it, it's good for you.

*Frozen Produce: Although I use fresh produce whenever possible, frozen fruits and vegetables still possess a good portion of the vitamins and minerals found in their fresh counterparts. The only drawback to me is they seem to quickly lose their crispness during cooking. I always keep a few bags of different vegetables in the freezer, especially for use in the winter when my favorites are not abundantly available.

*Celery Seed: Celery seeds are a great addition to soups, salads and many other dishes. They have been used for many years as a diuretic, for lowering blood pressure and for their stress-reducing effects. If your blood pressure is through the roof celery seed may be of help. Though I prefer cooking with celery, when I don't have some around I just pop in these little healthful seeds.

* Quinoa: Found by the Incas a few thousand years ago when they discovered it was edible, quinoa is often mistaken for a grain but is actually a gluten-free seed. Loaded with tons of healthy components and rich in protein and fiber, it possesses lots of vitamins and that all-important magnesium. Quinoa is delicious and easy to prepare, and makes a wonderful change from rice, couscous or pasta. For a stellar side dish, dress it up with veggies, healthy spices and fresh herbs.

* Canned Mackerel: Nutritionists advise at least two

servings of fish per week to get our adequate dose of omega-3. I usually prepare fish about three times a week, but sometimes the prices are so high that I cut back a little. For those times, I keep several cans of canned mackerel in the pantry. These little fish may have a bad rap but they taste great and are loaded with omega-3 and magnesium. For a quick and tasty lunch I serve the mackerel on a lettuce bed with a side of veggies and a squeeze of lemon.

Chapter 7: A Grab Bag of Healthy Ideas

I wrote this book to share what I've learned about mental, physical and emotional well-being, so in one sense you can consider me your cheerleader. Perhaps many of you have already heard much of what I have presented here, but have yet to personally reap the benefits of organic foods, daily exercise and some of the other disciplines covered. I have tried them all and credit them with keeping me healthy. My hope is that you will be inspired to do the same and sprinkle bits of my advice into your daily life, helping you to feel good and commit to feeling even better.

Far too many drugs are prescribed for problems that can often be solved naturally without suffering the debilitating side effects common to so many drugs. Certainly some people need to take specific, targeted drugs in order to survive and live comfortably. But for those common complaints that seem to appear in all of us as we age, simple changes in lifestyle can be the fix.

My husband and I are close in age, both in our seventies. Neither of us takes any prescription drugs, just specific supplements. We ride our racing bikes almost every day, tackling some challenging hills. I am 5' 6" tall and weigh 125 pounds, as I have for my entire adult life. I'm still a size 6. Believe me, I'm not boasting, just hoping to set an example and show you my path.

While doing research for this book, I was amazed at the enormous amount of information that has been published on health-related topics. There are books written by experts with multiple degrees and others by people who have lived with certain problems and overcome them through trial and error. Much of what is out there is helpful and insightful, but sticking with new ways of life is still a daunting challenge. So many of us become enamored with a new diet or exercise program, achieving moderate success and even staying healthy for a short period of time. However, too often after a few weeks we slip back into old habits.

The simple truth is, success and change come in bits and pieces. I can guarantee you will not wake up one day and think, "Wow, everything I've tried has worked!" In fact, the change can be so gradual, it may take you months to realize you that you're feeling better, have dropped a few pounds and have lowered your blood pressure.

So here is my challenge to you: Try one new thing that you've read about in this book every day, for the next 365 days. Even trying one new thing each *week* can help you create a steadily growing habit that will net amazing results. And please know that I am wishing you the best of luck from afar.

Building lifelong habits

Our habits are the mainstay of our existence. We develop daily habits early on, from brushing our teeth and taking showers to feeding the cat or making the coffee. We may make our bed every day on automatic pilot. When we decide to make a change or add something new to our routine, it's not done overnight. According to experts it takes three weeks to get rid of a habit and three weeks to develop a new one. Food is no exception.

Though we may not realize it, eating certain foods at certain times is habitual behavior, some of it good and some not so good.

My eating and exercising habits have been with me for years, with occasional changes and modifications. Sometimes the weather, travel or other changes in our lives will modify our habits for a limited period of time. I have noticed if I don't exercise or eat as healthfully as I usually do it is a challenge getting back on track. But if your commitment to health is strong, you'll develop new and positive habits.

Making better choices

One thing that most of us are fortunate to have in life is the freedom of choice, even if the outcome resulting from our choice is out of our hands. Many of us reflect on past decisions with either a pat on the back for making a wise choice or a stern talking-to for doing the wrong thing.

Perhaps you have made a choice to eat healthier. Let's say you've decided to give up that sweet roll for breakfast and instead have a slice of toast with peanut butter. Sounds good — but is it really? Eating white bread with commercially processed peanut butter may be no better than the sweet roll. Whole grain bread and natural peanut butter are a different story. See where I'm going with this? It's important to recognize when you have replaced a bad habit with a really good one.

Eating out

Face it: restaurant dining is part of our social landscape. We go out to with friends and family to celebrate a special occasion, or maybe just to enjoy a night off from cooking and cleaning up. But what happens to your good intentions of eating healthy when you're faced with that fancy menu? The bad news is that most restaurant food is made to taste good and get you coming back for more. To that end, much of it contains too much fat, sugar and salt. But take heart; there is hardly any situation -- be it a special restaurant, a dinner party at a friend's home, a fancy wedding -- where you cannot make a healthful food choice, though it may not be to your liking.

It's tempting to tell yourself, "Just for tonight I will eat what I want and I promise I'll be good tomorrow." If you go out for dinner only occasionally, it's fine to just chalk it up as a rare night out and order a favorite dish regardless of calories or fat content. And if you've been diligent about staying healthy in your own kitchen, you do deserve a treat. However, for those who habitually eat out several times a week it's important to lay down some ground rules.

*Healthy Restaurant Rules:

1. Don't go hungry.
Before going out, drink a glass of tomato juice or a cup of warm broth. This helps stave off the immediate hunger that arises when you first encounter the enticing smells in the restaurant.

2. Beware the breadbasket.
Bread, and the accompanying butter or dipping olive oil, is always an issue. I will indulge if it is absolutely my favorite crusty French bread or popovers, a rare treat and my favorite. Otherwise I simply ask the server to remove the breadbasket.

3. Dip into dressings.

If you order a salad, ask for the dressing to be served on the side. Then, instead of pouring it on, dip your fork into some dressing before you take some salad. You'll get the flavor but far fewer calories.

4. Be a Plain Jane.

When choosing a main course, avoid thick or creamy sauces and order something recognizable, prepared as plainly as possible.

5. Ask for veggies instead.
When rice, potatoes and vegetables are offered, ask your server for double the veggie order and pass on the starch.

6. Skip dessert.
If you feel you absolutely must indulge, just order one dessert for the whole group, with extra forks. You'll be surprised at how just a taste can satisfy your sweet tooth.

*Ethnic Foods:
Italian restaurants may be your favorite. Instead of pasta, order veal, chicken or beef with a tomato-based sauce.

Chinese and Thai restaurants can fool you. At first glance the menu looks pretty healthful, but be aware that there is a ton of sugar hiding in most Asian dishes. Ask your server to suggest something that is not fried or heavily salted.

Mexican food is growing in popularity, along with peoples' waistbands. I like it well enough, but steer clear of the enchiladas and other calorie-laden dishes. I will often order fajitas and eat the meat, onions and peppers, leaving the tortillas on my plate.

Stay away from sugar

There was a time when I indulged in sweet desserts far too often, until I realized sugar's addictive qualities. Even now, if I splurge and have a small piece of cake I'm craving sugar the next day. We all know it is not good for our bodies – or our figures—but addiction is hard to overcome no matter what the substance. I have friends who can't go a whole day without eating something sweet, and fruit simply won't satisfy that nagging sweet tooth. Fortunately the natural sweetness of fruit does the trick for me. Give it a try!

Think about finding other ways to cut back on your sugar intake, especially if you experience extreme highs and lows after eating some. Your commitment starts at the grocery store: keeping sugary treats out of your cupboard is the best way to start reducing your sugar intake.

Why organic?

When it comes to buying food, *organic* is a buzzword these days. Several years ago it was difficult to find organic produce, whereas today most grocery stores have a huge selection marked organic. I do buy organic when it is affordable and available, but I am not obsessed like many people are. My feeling is that if you wash your fruits and vegetables thoroughly you will remove most of the pesticides. I use a special veggie and fruit wash regardless if the produce is organic or not.

Sadly, much of our soil over the past years has become depleted, meaning there are fewer vitamins and minerals in the food being grown commercially today. That may explain why growing your own produce has become so popular. Even having a small garden with herbs and a few easy to grow vegetables can add a lot to your good health. Besides, there is something very spiritual about growing your own vegetables. Despite the poor soil where we live in Arizona, I went ahead and started several small pots and now grow my own herbs, tomatoes, peppers and okra.

The term *organic* does not only refer to produce. Organic grass-fed beef has become popular among people who want absolutely no chemicals to enter their systems, even from the foods that their food has eaten! And these days most chicken purveyors do not use antibiotics, while others don't inject their birds with hormones. I look for hormone-free chickens and always buy organic when it's on sale. And honestly, organic chickens really do taste better.

Buying organic is a choice, and naturally your budget comes into play as these choices always cost more. However, the following fruits and veggies are best grown organically due to their high pesticide residue.

apples
strawberries
grapes
celery
peaches
spinach
sweet bell peppers
imported nectarines
cucumbers
cherry tomatoes
imported snap peas
potatoes

The following foods have very little pesticide residue as they either grow low to the ground or are protected by skin coverage.

onions
avocados
mangos

sweet peas
kiwi fruit
sweet corn
asparagus
broccoli
papaya
cabbage
Brussels sprouts
pineapple

High vs. low fat

I remember when being on a low-fat diet was the way to go to stay healthy and lose weight. Things have changed and fat is back with a vengeance. However the attitude about different fats and oils has also changed. For non-fat and low-fat products to stay fresh and have flavor, they are augmented with sugar, other harmful additives or just plain water. Sure they have fewer calories, but they're also not good for you.

It's important to remember that eating *healthy* fats is beneficial to your health. When I buy dairy products they are full-fat and if possible, organic. If you are concerned about the calories, it's better just to cut back your portion sizes than to buy the low-fat version.

Exercise

There are many opinions floating around about exercising. Some experts advise working out no more than 90 minutes total for the week. The most important thing is doing what feels good to you. Before embarking on an exercise program be sure to check with your health provider, particularly if you have been living a sedentary lifestyle. You don't have to join the latest craze; walking has always been a wonderful way to get moving. It doesn't require any expensive equipment besides a good pair of supportive shoes to reap the emotional rewards of being out in nature.

My husband and I ride bicycles which we have been doing most of our lives. Biking is easy on the joints and has the bonus of getting you outside in the fresh air. We also work out four or five days a week. If you aren't up for going to a gym, make sure to move around as much as you are physically able. Gardening, cleaning and just walking around the house all count.

If you spend a lot of time at the computer like I do, make sure to stand up at least once every hour. Walk around and do some stretching to avoid sore muscles, and give your eyes a rest too. The most important thing about exercising is if you're having fun while you're doing it, it will surely become part of your daily routine.

* **Weight Training:** Check online or with a professional trainer for some simple exercises you

can do with weights. To get started you can use just 1-pound weights to maintain strength and support good bone health, increasing the weight as you become stronger. I lift weights while sitting at the computer to avoid back strain. This is a simple way to keep our bones strong as we age, requiring very little time each day.

* **Yoga:** Yoga has been around for literally centuries, and its popularity continues to grow. I personally have gone to yoga classes off and on throughout my adult years. It helps improve your muscle tone, balance, mobility and flexibility. For me, the best part of any yoga class was the last several minutes where you close your eyes, take a deep breath and rest. Recently, writing about yoga has inspired me to head back to class. Today there are many special yoga classes sprouting up for seniors, involving a more gentle way to achieve the same goals.

* **Facial Exercise:** We exercise our bodies to stay in shape, so why not our faces? For me, doing whatever I can to look and feel my best is important. To that end, I do facial exercises almost every day. They are less expensive cheaper and certainly less invasive than plastic surgery. Do I look 20 years younger? Probably not. Still, I have a pretty firm jawline that makes me think they're accomplishing something!

I can promise that if you start doing these exercises daily you will eventually notice an improvement in the contours of your face. There are many programs available online, but I have found that one called Facial Magic works best for me. Check it out!

The mind-body connection

* Reiki: Reiki is a Japanese technique that can reduce stress and support healing. The Reiki practitioner can lay hands on specific points on the body or just put their hands several inches above the area. The theory is that "life force energy" flows through us and can be aided with the Reiki treatment. If one's "life force energy" is low there is a chance the person is more open to getting sick or feeling stressed out.

Reiki has been practiced for centuries for many types of healing, and it is still popular today to reduce stress, support healing and work in coordination with medical procedures.

Several years ago I had a very sore knee and I had a friend who was a Reiki practitioner. She offered to give me a few Reiki treatments and of course I said yes not having a clue what she was talking about. After 4 treatments my knee felt great and still does.

There are three degrees of Reiki Practitioners: Reiki 1 Practitioner, Reiki 11 Advanced Practitioner and Reiki Master. I am currently a Reiki 11 practitioner and soon will be a Reiki Master. When you receive your

Reiki 11 practitioner certification you can work remote on people. I treated my husband remotely from class and he was home. He felt very warm afterwards and claimed his back felt better. This may sound very strange to you, but it works. Since that time I have worked on several people remote and they have had amazing results.

* **Tapping:** Tapping, also known as EFT or Emotional Freedom Technique, combines the art of ancient Chinese acupressure with modern psychology. Using your fingertips, you tap on one of nine specific pressure points and direct your energy to whatever is bothering you, while making a positive statement such as, "I deeply and completely love and accept myself." You can find charts on the Internet that easily demonstrate how this is done. Better yet, find a class at a local college and get involved more deeply.

After you have mastered this exercise, you can easily move on to reducing problems that are stressing you. I found after doing this only one time I reduced my stress and anxiety by almost half. The more I repeated this exercise the more peaceful I felt.
And the best part is that you can do this anywhere and it doesn't take very long.

* **Massage:** Massage is a general term referring to the manipulation of your skin, muscles, tendons and ligaments. It is generally relaxing and calming and can treat a variety of problems, including anxiety,

headaches, insomnia and sports injuries. You may want to try more than one type of massage, which differ in the amount of pressure applied. Swedish Massage is gentle, while Deep Massage is slower and more forceful. Trigger Point Massage concentrates on specific muscle fibers.

Be sure to ask your health practitioner which kind is best for your particular situation. And bear in mind, there are times when having any massage is ill-advised. For example, if you have a fever, feel dizzy or nauseated, have bruises, wounds or sunburn, or were recently involved in a car accident, it may be unsafe for you. Even some medications may preclude your having a massage. If you are uncertain whether you should or shouldn't, check with your health provider beforehand.

* Foot Massage: A reflexology (foot) massage is very healthful and relaxing. Because the pressure points on the bottom of the foot relate to different organs and parts of your body, a single reflexology session can reduce anxiety, diminish pain, improve blood flow and decrease high blood pressure. Check online for complete instructions and diagrams showing the important pressure points of the foot.

Best of all, it's simple to do. To lessen depression and anxiety, pinch your big toe with the thumb and first finger and hold for about 10 seconds. Do this with both feet. Next, try pressing the indentation just below your middle toe for several seconds and then take a deep breath. This is can help regulate your blood pressure. Finally, massage your feet from heel to toe for about five to ten minutes just before going to bed. I do this massage several times a week and I have found it to relax me into a restful sleep. Plus my feet feel good!

* **Meditation:** With so many books, podcasts, websites and magazines devoted to it, meditation has been portrayed as something quite complicated and taking years to master. This is simply not true. Meditation can be a simple act and one that will quickly relieve stress and relax your mind and body. Try it and see.

Find a quiet corner of your house, then simply sit back in a comfy chair. (Just doing this much could challenge many of you.) Next, simply breathe in and out, focusing on your breath. Breathe in, hold and exhale, working at breathing with your abdomen. But that's just one way. Many people breathe through the mouth and focus on a specific mantra, or short group of soothing words. I find it easier to count breaths. I breathe in for four seconds, hold for eight seconds, and slowly exhale for seven.

I usually meditate between five and ten minutes a day because that works for me. Meditation takes a lot of discipline to give yourself a few minutes off from your routine, but the results are amazing. Soon enough you will feel less stressed and feel more in control of your thoughts, rather than having them control you.

*** Tai Chi and Qigong:** These ancient Chinese practices are basically exercises and techniques for achieving and maintaining greater balance, flexibility and peacefulness. Qigong is less vigorous than Tai Chi for those who have some challenges in moving and flexing. There are many classes available all over the country, and generally people can do these gentle exercises well into old age.
I recently attended a Qigong class that included a bit of yoga and meditation. This was my first time doing Qigong and I found it easy, with no challenging moves. I felt great afterwards, and once back home I was pleased that I could stay quiet and meditate for thirty minutes.

A few extras

*** Oil Pulling:** More than 1,000 years old, oil pulling is part of ancient Ayurvedic holistic health practices. The leading purpose of it is to rid the mouth of bacteria and toxins and whiten your teeth. Today it is controversial among health experts; many feel it has little benefit while others insist it does no harm. Personally, I have seen it work wonders. Here's how it's done: Swish about a tablespoon of coconut, sunflower or sesame oil in your mouth for about ten minutes, then spit it out.

While there is little noteworthy research on this activity, I did find many anecdotal claims of it having significant benefit. My husband, who sees a dentist quarterly for a cleaning, reluctantly agreed to try this practice for one week. At his next dental appointment the hygienist was amazed by the improved condition of his teeth and declared his usual deep cleaning unnecessary.

The buildup of bacteria in your mouth causes not just periodontal disease but also negatively impacts the entire body, since toxins travel throughout your organs. Oil pulling is just another way to work at staying healthy as we age.

* **Diet Soda:** Diet soda may seem out of place among all these healthful suggestions and ideas. However, I feel so passionately about *not* drinking diet soda that I had to mention it here. Our national addiction to diet soda is as great as the addiction to sugar. Diet soda tricks the brain into thinking it is getting sugar, thus increasing your desire for sugar. And since it contains no calories, you are more apt to eat more. If you stop drinking diet soda your body will thank you in many ways, including with better kidney function and bone health.

* **Glycemic Index:** The glycemic index ranks foods from 1 to 100 based on their effect on blood-sugar levels. Though important information for all of us, it is

essential for diabetics in order to keep their blood sugar in a safe range. Foods below 55 on the index are considered low and foods above 69 are considered high. There are many charts online showing complete lists of foods, from the highest to the lowest on the glycemic index. Here are some low-glycemic foods:

asparagus
avocados
olive oil
most nuts
most legumes
apples
kiwis
blueberries
strawberries

Here are some examples foods that are high on the glycemic index:
bananas
crackers
white potatoes
sodas
bread
raisins
dates
pastries

***Antioxidants:** It seems like we're always hearing about the benefits of antioxidants. A complicated subject, it can be better understood in simple terms. Basically, our bodies are beaten up daily by "free radicals" such as pollutants, unhealthy foods and a variety of drugs, often with dire results like disease and debilitating conditions. Help arrives in the form of specific antioxidants found in foods as well as supplements that target and protect all parts of the body. Antioxidants benefit the body by neutralizing and sometimes removing the free radicals, thus creating a stronger immune system.

Here are some of the top antioxidant foods:
dark chocolate
artichokes
kidney beans
cranberries
blackberries
cilantro
green tea
cloves
cinnamon
turmeric
cumin
basil
ginger
thyme
garlic
cayenne pepper

Top antioxidant herbs:
cloves
cinnamon
turmeric

cumin
basil
ginger
thyme
garlic
cayenne pepper

Top antioxidant essential oils:
lavender
Frankincense
basil oil
wintergreen
cypress
rose
peppermint

Top antioxidant supplements:
lutein (eyes)
vitamin E (skin and eyes)
vitamin C (colds, flu and skin)
astaxanthin (eyes, joints energy)
selenium
quercetin (found in berries, leafy greens or supplements)
glutathione (a booster of other antioxidants and vitamins)

Now it's your turn!

We have reached the end of the book and the start of your personal commitment.

I have tried most of the health and beauty recipes described in these pages, and have heard from friends how much better they feel after enacting some of my suggestions. Now it's your turn! Try some of my recipes, follow up with some exercise and a healthier lifestyle, and be ambitious in researching a few of the ideas that are new to you.

To my knowledge there are no foods, supplements, exercises or creams that will create a younger body. Food will surely nourish you, supplements will support your body and improve your cognitive skills and memory, and plastic surgery can create a younger-looking face for a period of time. But the only way to feel better and enjoy improved health is to take full responsibility for your actions and commit to a healthier lifestyle. If you start now to make slow and deliberate changes, before you know it you'll feel better, have more energy, and find more peace in life.

Starting today, make some changes:

Try some new spices and herbs in your cooking.
Switch to healthy oils for cooking.
Add one serving of vegetables a day.
Start a new habit of walking with just a walk around the block.

Make your own toothpaste or hand cream.
Try one new healthful recipe a week from the recipe section.
Add a supplement that supports a condition you may have.
Experiment with one relaxation technique you have never tried.
Start working out with 1-pound weights.
Do more reading on topics that interested you in this book.
Share all of this with a partner to keep you both on track.

Biography

Carol Stanley lives in Arizona with her husband Jim and their 13-year-old cat, Elwood. The author of three other books, one a bestseller, she's always got something cooking, be it a delicious healthy meal or some natural skin care potions or cleaning products. To stay in great shape, Carol enjoys daily bike riding and hiking, with some yoga and weight training thrown in. When it's time to relax, she opts for reading, playing the keyboard, painting tote bags and playing poker.

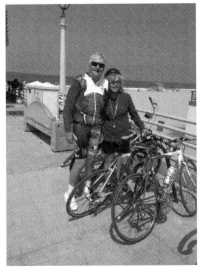

Surely the youngest senior you'll ever meet, Carol would love to help all of her peers stay healthy and learn how they can feel better every day.

She welcomes your questions and comments at: *carolstanley1@yahoo.com.*

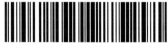

Made in the USA
Columbia, SC
06 December 2017